DIAGNOSTIC
Picture
in Clinical

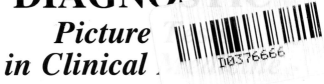

1

G S J Chessell, Dip Ed Tech.
Coordinator, Medical Learning Resources Group,
University of Aberdeen

M J Jamieson, MRCP
Lecturer, Department of Therapeutics and Clinical
Pharmacology, University of Aberdeen

R A Morton, MSc
Director, Department of Medical Illustration,
University of Aberdeen

J C Petrie, FRCP
Reader, Department of Therapeutics and Clinical
Pharmacology, University of Aberdeen; Honorary
Consultant Physician, Aberdeen Teaching
Hospitals.

H M A Towler, MRCP
Lecturer, Department of Medicine,
University of Aberdeen.

Wolfe Publishing Ltd

© The University of Aberdeen 1984
Published by Wolfe Medical Publications Ltd 1984
Printed by Grafos, Arte Sobre Papel, Barcelona, Spain
Volume 1 ISBN 0 7234 0848 3
Volume 2 ISBN 0 7234 0849 1
Volume 3 ISBN 0 7234 0850 5
Volume 4 ISBN 0 7234 0851 3

Reprinted 1985, 1987, 1989, 1991, 1992

For a full list of Wolfe Medical Atlases, plus
forthcoming titles and details of our surgical,
dental and veterinary Atlases, please write to
Wolfe Publishing Limited,
Brook House,
2-16 Torrington Place
London WC1E 7LT

PREFACE

This is volume one of a four-volume series. The aim is to test diagnostic skills over a wide range of clinical problems. Questions which may feature in examinations or in clinical practice are posed in an attempt to stimulate the undergraduate or postgraduate reader to undertake further reading.

The pictures in this new series have been selected from the clinical slide library in the Department of Medical Illustration, University of Aberdeen. The books have been produced against a background of experience gained over the last 10 years in the compilation for local use of over 2,000 self-assessment examples. The local exercise was coordinated through the Medical Learning Resources Group of the Faculty of Medicine, University of Aberdeen, in collaboration with many of the clinicians in the Aberdeen Teaching Hospitals.

We hope that the books will be of interest to all who are committed to their own continuing medical education. We would welcome comment on individual questions and answers.

GSJC, MJJ, RAM, JCP, HMAT.

Although numbering is sequential, each volume in the series is unique, containing a balanced selection of diagnostic examples, and thus may be used independently.

ACKNOWLEDGEMENTS

We wish to acknowledge the invaluable contribution of Dr Anthony Hedley, now Professor of Community Medicine, University of Glasgow, who was the instigator of the self-assessment programme on which these books are based. We would also like to acknowledge the cooperation of all patients, secretarial and technical staff, in particular the staff of the Department of Medical Illustration, who have contributed in one way or another to the preparation of these volumes, and Mrs Margaret Doverty who typed the manuscript.

We would particularly like to thank the following colleagues for contributing material for the books:

Dr D R Abramovich, Mr A Adam, Mr A K Ah-See, Dr D J G Bain, Dr L S Bain, Dr K Bartlett, Dr A P Bayliss, Dr B Bennett, Miss F M Bennett, Dr P Best, Dr P D Bewsher, Mr C Birchall, Mr C T Blaiklock, Dr L J Borthwick, Mr P L Brunnen, Dr P W Brunt, Dr J Calder, Professor A G M Campbell, Dr B Carrie, Dr P Carter, Dr G R D Catto, Mr R B Chesney, Dr N Clark, Mr P B Clarke, Mr A I Davidson, Dr R J L Davidson, Dr A A Dawson, Mr W B M Donaldson, Professor A S Douglas, Dr A W Downie, Dr C J Eastmond, Mr J Engeset, Dr N Edward, Dr J K Finlayson, Dr J R S Finnie, Mr A V Foote, Dr N G Fraser, Mr R J A Fraser, Dr J A R Friend, Dr D B Galloway, Mr J M C Gibson, Dr D Hadley, Dr J E C Hern, Dr A W Hutcheon, Dr T A Jeffers, Dr A W Johnston, Mr P F Jones, Dr A C F Kenmure, Mr I R Kernohan, Dr A S M Khir, Mr J Kyle, Dr J S Legge, Mr McFadzean, Dr E McKay, Mr J McLauchlan, Mr K A McLay, Professor M MacLeod, Dr R A Main, Mr Mather, Mr N A Matheson, Mr J D B Miller, Mr S S Miller, Mr K L G Mills, Dr N A G Mowat, Mr I F K Muir, Dr L E Murchison, Mr W J Newlands, Mr J G Page, Professor R Postlethwaite, Dr J M Rawles, Mr P K Ray, Mr C R W Rayner, Professor A M Rennie, Mr A G R Rennie, Dr J A N Rennie, Dr O J Robb, Dr H S Ross, Dr G Russell, Dr D S Short, Dr P J Smail, Dr C C Smith, Professor G Smith, Dr L Stankler, Mr J H Steyn, Professor J M Stowers, Dr G H Swapp, Mr J Wallace, Professor W Walker, Dr S J Watt, Dr J Weir, Dr J Webster, Dr M I White, Dr F W Wigzell, Dr M J Williams, Mr L C Wills, Dr L A Wilson, Mr H A Young.

1

This thirty-five year old woman complained of tinnitus in her left ear. Clinical examination revealed an absent gag reflex and weakness of the soft palate, sternomastoid and trapezius on the left.

a What abnormality is seen in the middle ear?

b What is the most likely diagnosis?

c How should this condition be treated?

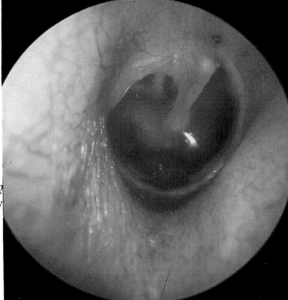

1

2 This is the bone-marrow aspirate smear of a thirty year old woman. Three months after returning from a holiday which involved travelling overland from Nepal to Turkey, she has developed biphasic diurnal fever, anaemia, splenomegaly, and recurrent epistaxis.

a What abnormality is present and which diagnosis does it indicate?

b Which vector is responsible for transmission of this disease?

c What drug therapy is appropriate?

2

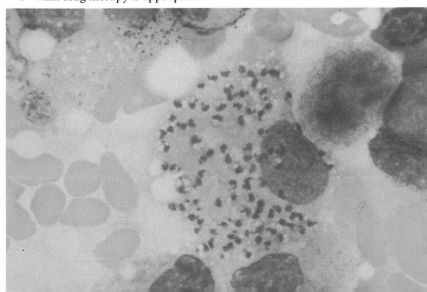

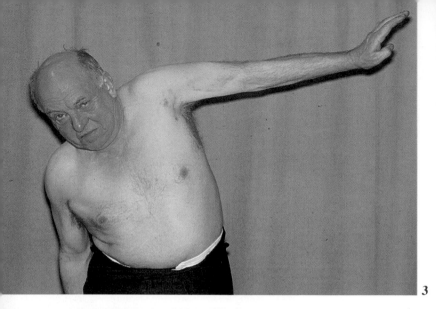

3

3 This patient is unable to initiate abduction of the left arm. He is, however. able to maintain abduction of the passively abducted arm, as seen here. What is the diagnosis?

4 a What is the likely cause of this patient's painful knee?
  b What common name is given to this condition?
  c Is the knee joint likely to be involved?

4

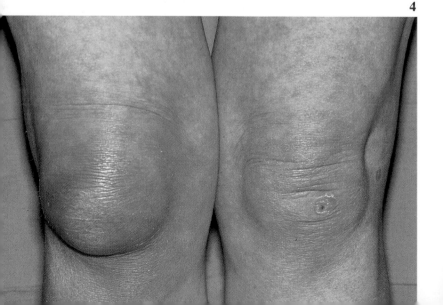

5 This seventy year old patient gives a two month history of temporal headaches. He has been aware of tenderness of the scalp, especially when combing his hair.

a What diagnosis does the history suggest?

b Which symptoms and which sign are regarded as pathognomonic of this disorder?

c What abnormalities are seen in the picture?

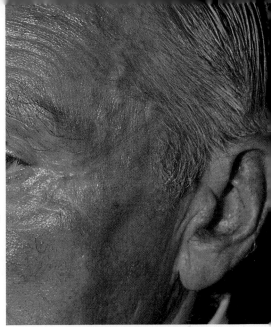

6 This patient is bedridden because of severe disseminated sclerosis. He has recently developed mild dependent oedema associated with heavy proteinuria (more than three grammes/day) and hypoalbuminaemia.

a What is the likely cause of the lesions seen around his right buttock?

b How might this explain his proteinuria?

c What investigation would you choose to establish the diagnosis?

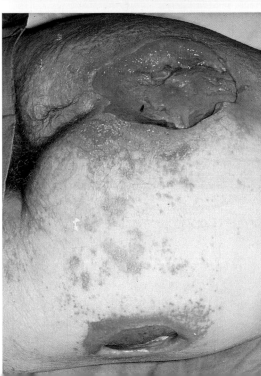

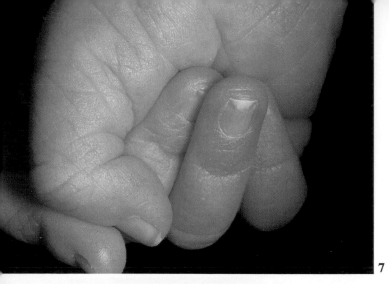

7

7 and 8 These abnormalities are characteristic of a chromosomal disorder.
   a What name is given to the foot abnormality?
   b What is the chromosomal disorder?
   c What is the prognosis of this disorder?

8

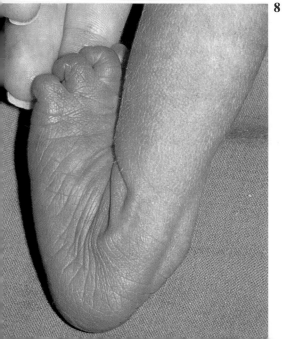

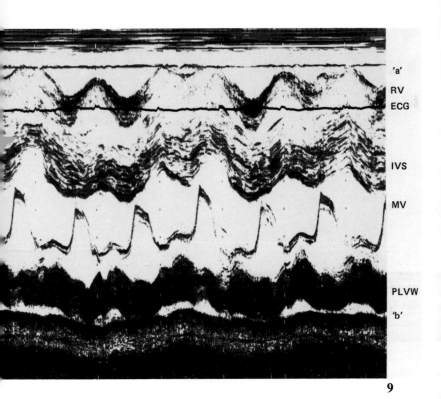

9

RV   — right ventricular wall
ECG   — electrocardiogram
IVS   — interventricular septum
MV   — mitral valve
PLVW — posterior left ventricular wall

This M-mode echocardiogram is from a fourteen year old boy with Hodgkin's disease.

a What is the cause of the echo-free spaces 'a' and 'b'?
b Which two other abnormalities are seen and what do these indicate?
c What urgent treatment may be necessary?

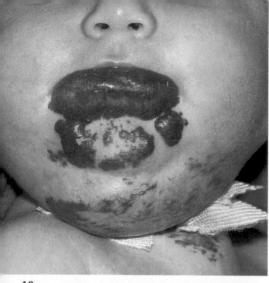

10 This lesion was not present at birth, but has gradually increased in size since then.
  a What is the lesion?
  b Give four reasons why specific treatment for such a lesion might be considered.

10
11

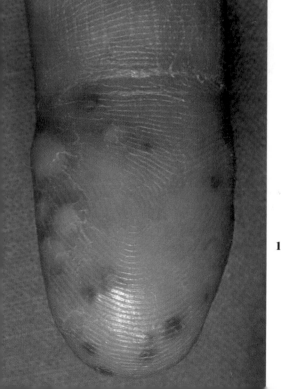

11 This nurse complains of painful lesions of her index finger.
  a What are these lesions?
  b What investigation is most helpful in establishing the diagnosis?

12

This patient complains of discomfort in his neck and axillae after drinking alcohol. He has recently become aware of a change in the appearance of his skin.

a What name is given to the abnormal skin appearance?

b What is the most likely underlying disorder?

c List three other diseases associated with a similar skin abnormality.

13

This patient's right pupil reacts to accommodation but not to light. The smaller left pupil reacts normally.

a What name is given to the abnormal pupillary response?

b This patient's pupillary reactions and appearances are typical of neurosyphilis — true or false?

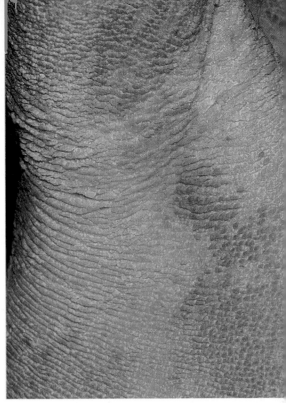

12

13

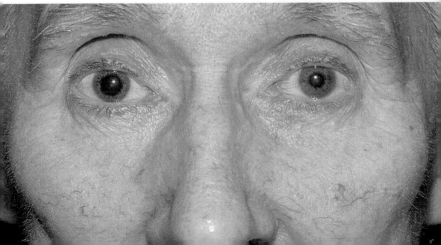

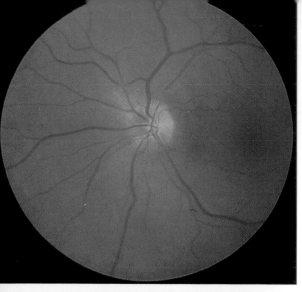

14

This patient complains of blurred vision. In order to focus on the retinal vessels, a normally-sighted examiner has to use a +10 dioptre lens.

a What visual abnormality does this indicate?

b What fundal abnormality is seen?

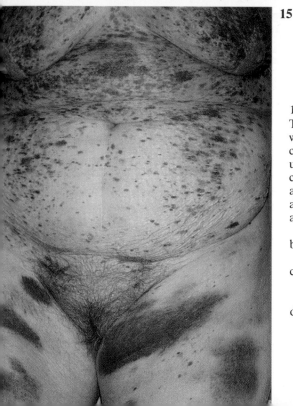

15

This seventy-six year old woman was treated with co-trimoxazole for a urinary tract infection. She complained of a sore throat a week before this appearance developed.

a What is the probable diagnosis?

b What clinical evidence would support this?

c What would bone marrow aspiration show?

d Which moiety of the co-trimoxazole is the likely culprit?

16, 17 and 18 This man presented with malaise, backache and deteriorating visual acuity. Haemoglobin was 8.8 g/dl and the erythrocyte sedimentation rate was 118mm. in the first hour.

a What radiological abnormalities are shown?

b What is the pathophysiology of the fundal appearance?

c What simple laboratory investigations are of great prognostic value?

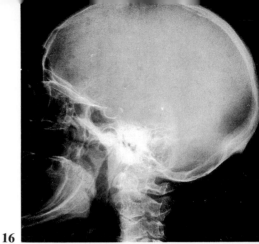

16

17

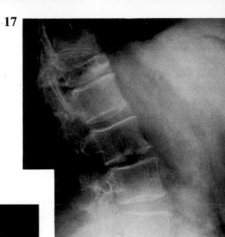

18

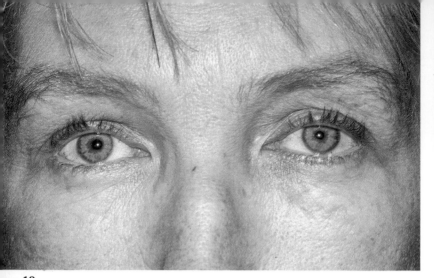

19

19 and 20 This patient's principal complaint is of pains across the shoulder girdle.

  a What abnormalities are seen in

     i)   her face?

     ii) her hands?

  b Suggest two possible diagnoses.

20

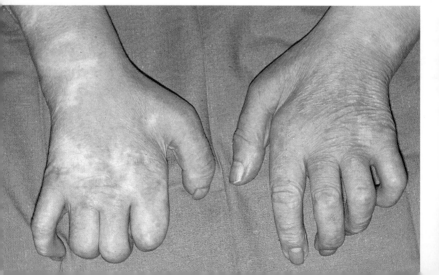

21 This patient has Graves'
disease.
  a Which ocular feature is
    demonstrated here?
  b How is this abnormality
    measured objectively?

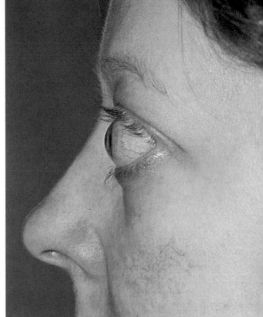

22 This patient has secondary
amenorrhoea.
  a What changes are seen
    in her right breast?
  b What is the diagnosis?
  c When did she have her
    last period?

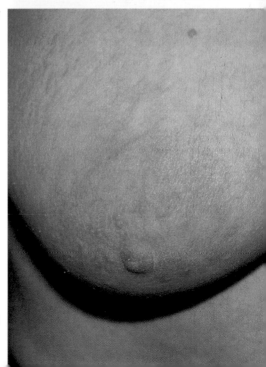

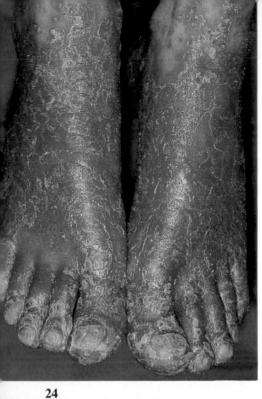

23

23 and 24 What metabolic
abnormality may these
patients have in common?

24

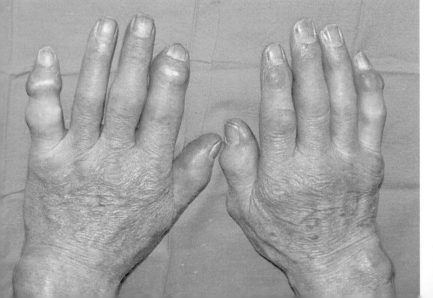

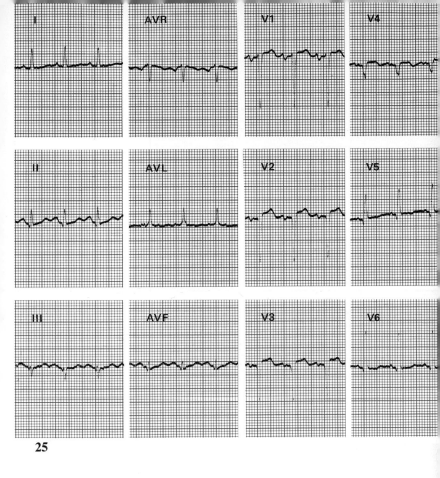

25

25 This sixty year old man had a myocardial infarction eight months ago. He has now developed refractory cardiac failure.

a What abnormalities are present?

b How may this explain his cardiac failure?

c What clinical signs may be present in addition to those of cardiac failure?

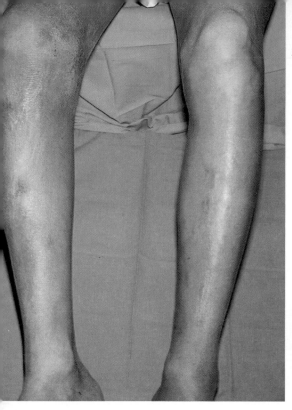

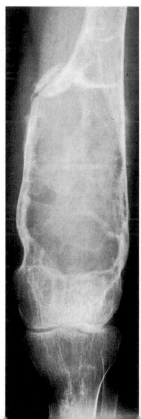

26 and 27 This patient complains of recurrent episodes of severe back pain, and, for years, of 'dragging' discomfort in his abdomen.

   a What abnormalities are seen:

      i) on the skin of his legs?

      ii) in the x-ray of femur?

   b What is the diagnosis?

   c What is likely to be found on abdominal examination?

   d Which biochemical abnormality is typical?

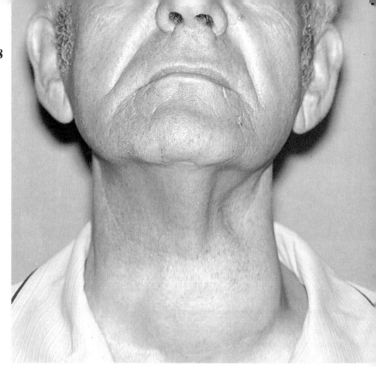

28 a Describe the principal abnormality shown.
   b Suggest three investigations which would help in making a diagnosis.
   c List three possible diagnoses.

29 This fifty-nine year old man with no previous history of bleeding
   problems presented with this appearance. The platelet count, bleeding
   time, thrombin time and prothrombin time were normal. The partial
   thromboplastin time was very long and not corrected by the addition of
   normal plasma or factor VIII.
   a What is the likely diagnosis?
   b In what conditions may this occur?

29

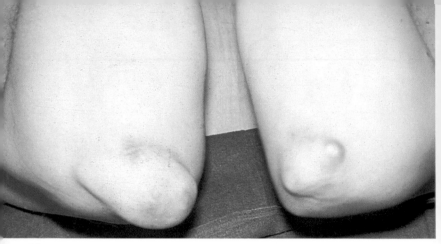

30

31

30 a What are these?
  b Where else do they occur?
  c What is their implication?

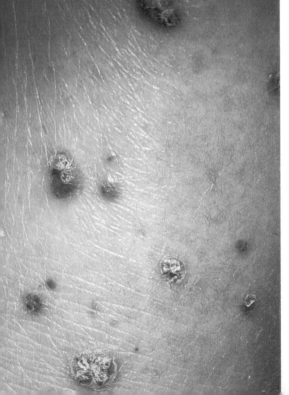

31

a What are these lesions?
b What forms of treatment are available for such lesions?

32 This male patient was referred because of short stature.
  a What features are shown?
  b What is the likely diagnosis?
  c How can this be confirmed?

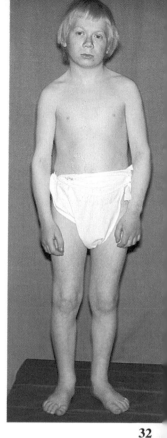

32

33

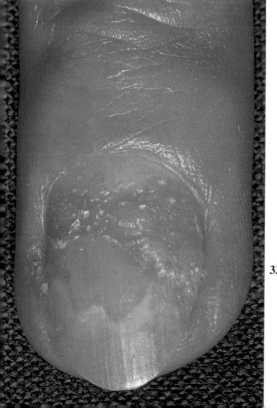

33 a What is the most likely diagnosis associated with the nail abnormalities shown?
  b What are the characteristic nail changes in this condition?

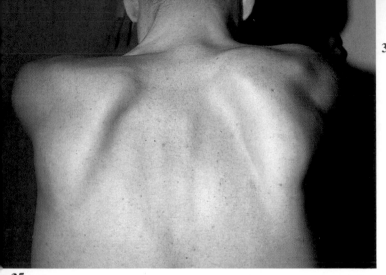

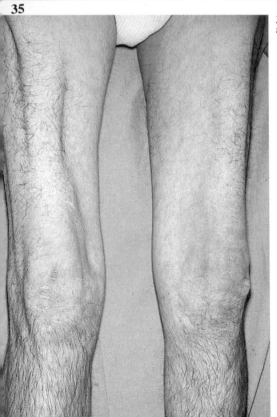

34
and 35 As a young man, this patient developed increasing weakness in his arms followed by proximal leg weakness. Limb-girdle dystrophy was diagnosed.
a Is he likely to be of low intelligence?
b Are the tendon reflexes normal in this condition?
c Is his life expectancy likely to be shortened?

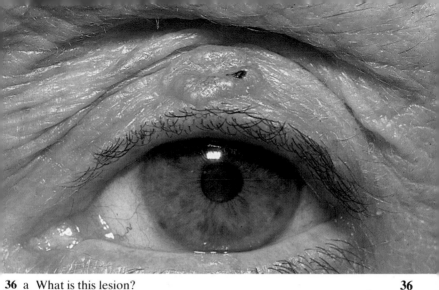

36 a What is this lesion?

    b What are the hazards of irradiating it?

    c What other therapies are available?

37

This man has a peripheral nerve lesion.

a Which nerve is principally affected?

b What unusual feature is present?

c How can this be explained?

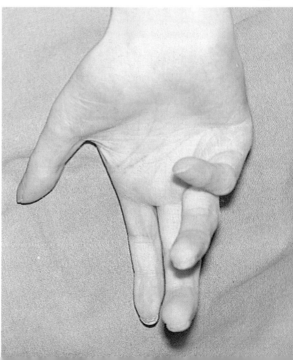

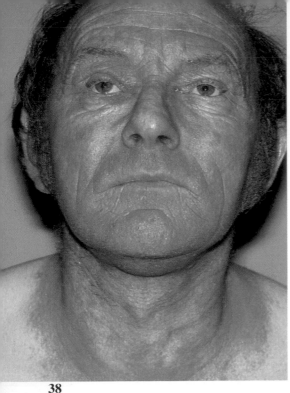

38
This patient is a maturity onset diabetic, and is hypertensive. His current regular medication includes amiloride, hydrochlorothiazide, nifedipine and chlorpropamide. Which of these drugs is/are most likely to be responsible for his skin rash?

39
This child suffers from chronic anaemia, recurrent infections and (until a recent surgical procedure) a severe bleeding tendency. During an acute respiratory illness the following results were obtained: Haemoglobin 3.5 g/dl. Blood film — hypochromia and considerable variation in red cell size, with red cell fragments; reticulocytosis

38
39

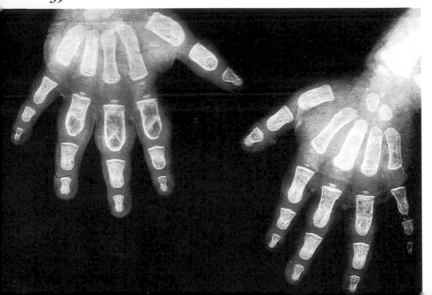

accompanied by large numbers of nucleated red cells; polymorph leucocytosis; platelet count normal.

a What abnormality is seen in the x-ray of the hands?

b What is the most likely diagnosis?

c Which surgical procedure was performed?

d Which complication of this procedure may have developed?

40

This lesion was present at birth and has slowly enlarged since.

a What is the likely diagnosis?

b What is the principal significance of such lesions?

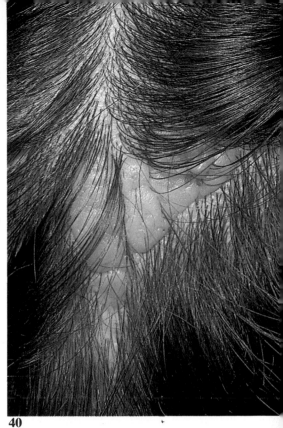

40

41 This patient's I.Q. is sixty.
a What ocular abnormality is seen?
b What is the diagnosis?

41

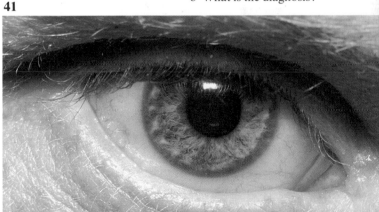

42

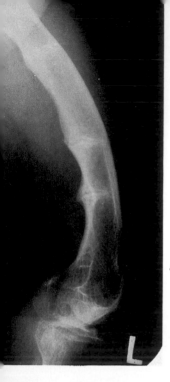

42 This patient is on regular treatment for epilepsy.
  a What abnormalities are seen in the x-ray of his femur?
  b What is the cause?
  c How does this relate to his epilepsy?

43

43
This patient has spent several years in Australia.
  a What is the most likely cause of the scalp abnormality seen?
  b What is the significance of this condition?

44

44
What is the most likely
cause of the asymptomatic
lesions seen on this
patient's thigh?

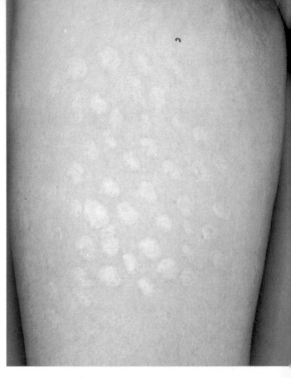

45

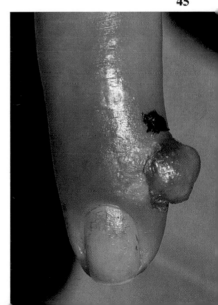

45 This lesion has increased in
   size rapidly over the past
   ten days. It has a tendency
   to bleed after minimal
   trauma.
   a What is the likely
     diagnosis?
   b What principal
     histological feature is
     typical?

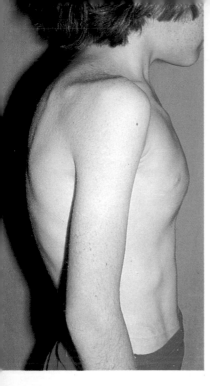

46 and 47

a What abnormality of this child's chest is seen?

b What is the most likely cause of his skin rash?

c List three ocular disorders associated with the skin condition.

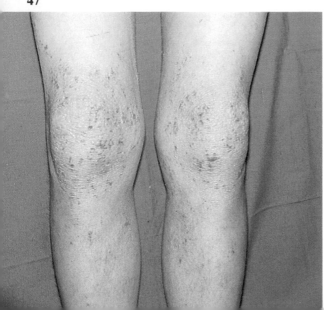

48

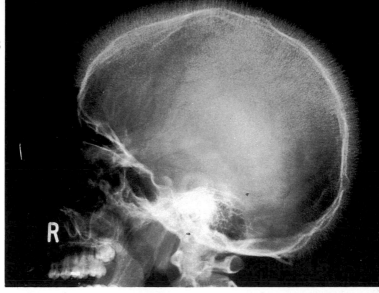

48 a What descriptive name is given to the radiological abnormality seen here?

    b What pathological process underlies the x-ray changes?

    c What is the most likely underlying condition?

49

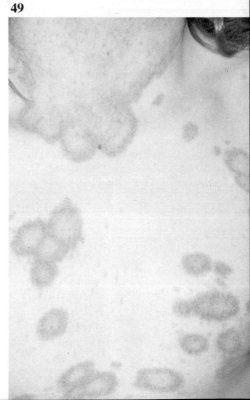

49 This patient presented with redness and itching of the axillae. Sensitivity to deodorant was diagnosed and a topical cream was prescribed. Application of the cream produced initial relief, but once therapy was stopped the itching returned and the rash became more widespread. Despite continued treatment with the cream the rash has continued to spread.

    a What name is given to this condition?

    b What is its cause?

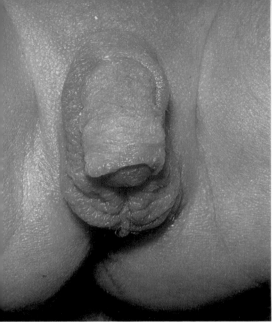

50

This baby's serum electrolytes include the following results. Sodium 120 mmol/l; potassium 5.6 mmol/l, bicarbonate 17 mmol/l; urea 9.0 mmol/l. Urinary sodium 40 mmol/l.

a What abnormality is demonstrated?
b Which diagnosis does the biochemistry and this appearance suggest?
c What is the likely biochemical defect?

50

51

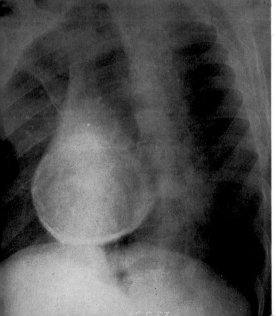

51

This patient presented with increasing tiredness and ankle oedema.

a What clinical abnormalities may be detected in the abdomen?
b What should be looked for on measuring her blood pressure?
c What may inspection of the jugular venous pulse reveal?
d What treatment is indicated?

52 and 53 This twenty-one year old male homosexual complained of a painful swollen left ankle. He had no urinary symptoms or recent alteration of bowel habit. Gram stain of joint aspirate showed intracellular Gram negative diplococci.

a What abnormalities are seen of his
  i) ankle?
  ii) feet?
b What is the most likely cause of his symptoms?
c How else should the diagnosis be established?

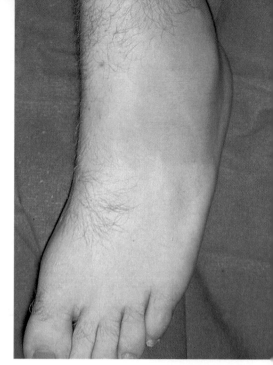

52

53

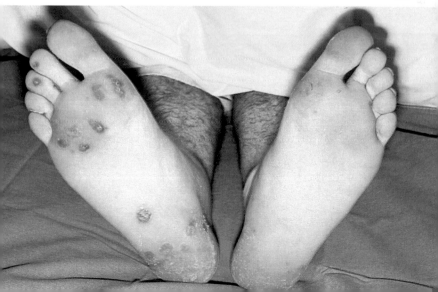

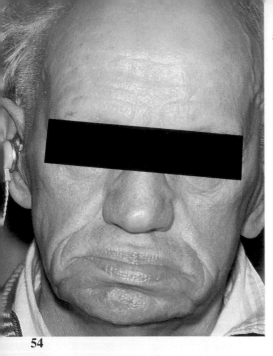

54 This patient has Huntington's chorea. His twenty-eight year old daughter is sixteen weeks pregnant.
  a What is the risk that her child will have the disorder?
  b How is the diagnosis established antenatally?
  c Which hepatic disorder is typically associated with this disease?

55 This child presented with fever, sore mouth and throat.
  a What abnormalities are shown on the anterior aspect of the tongue and thumb?
  b What is the likely diagnosis?
  c How could the oral and skin lesions be connected?

54

55

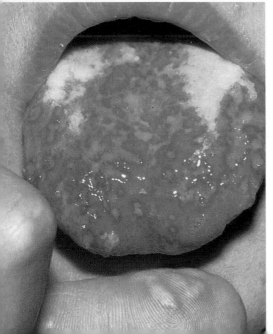

56 This patient suffers from chronic hepatocellular disease. Over the past two months he has lost three stones in weight and has complained of right upper quadrant pain. Abdominal examination reveals hepatomegaly, as delineated in pen, and an unusual auscultatory finding.
  a Suggest what the auscultatory finding may be.
  b What is your diagnosis?
  c List three factors which may predispose to this condition.

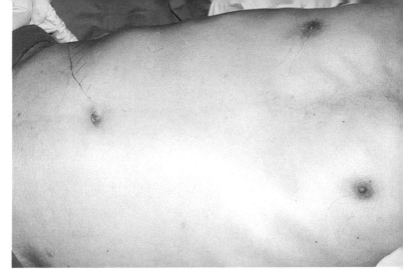

57 This patient was admitted following a haematemesis. Endoscopy revealed gastric erosions (probably related to recent ingestion of a nonsteroidal anti-inflammatory drug) but no other abnormality. She gave a history of four stones weight loss over the past two years but had no other abdominal symptoms. Haemoglobin was 8g/dl. The report on blood film was "hypochromic, microcytic anaemia. Howell Jolly bodies present". Barium meal showed no abnormality but flocculation of the barium column was observed on follow through.

a What is the most likely diagnosis?

b How does this explain the abnormal red cell features?

c What are the principal intestinal complications of this disorder?

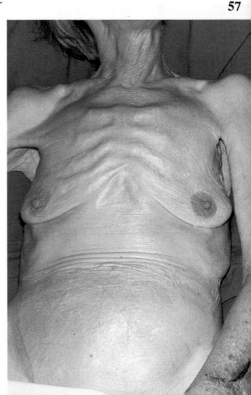

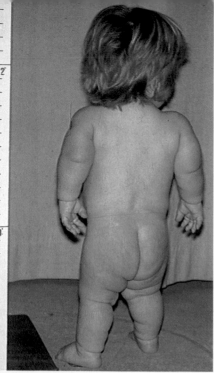

58

58 This child was born to normal parents.
   a What is this condition?
   b Which ossification process is abnormal?
   c What factor is associated with spontaneous cases of this disease?

59

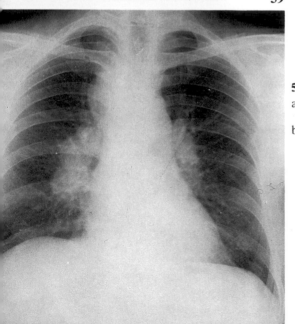

59
   a What abnormality is shown?
   b What feature suggests that this is non-neoplastic?

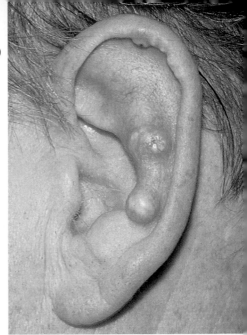

60 and 61

a What is the most likely nature of the abnormalities seen in this patient's ear and ring finger?

b In which tissue are such lesions never found?

c Suggest three means by which this disorder may impair renal function.

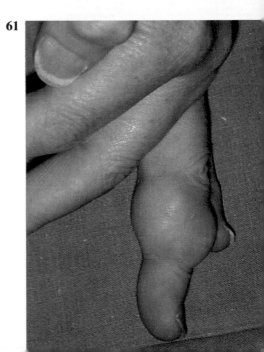

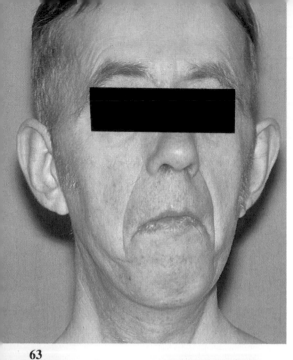

62
a What abnormal features are shown here?
b What is the likely diagnosis?

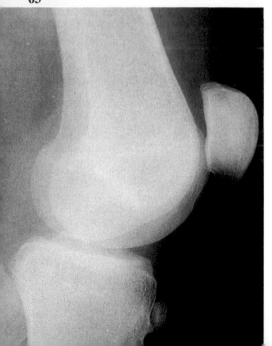

63 This young girl complains of recurrent pain in and swelling of the knee. What is the diagnosis?

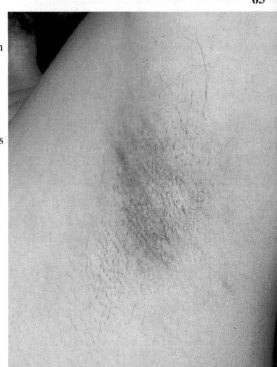

64

This patient presents with a history of weight loss, tiredness and blackouts.

a What two mucosal abnormalities are shown here?

b State the likely diagnosis.

c How can this be confirmed?

d List three important underlying causes of this disorder.

65

65

What should be suspected as the cause of this non-obese patient's iron deficiency anaemia?

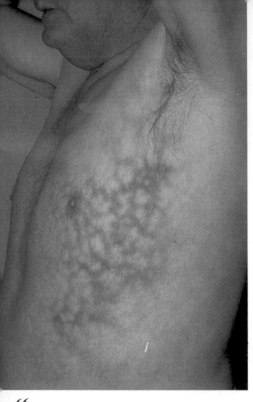

66 This patient complains of long-standing left sided chest pain.
  a What name is given to the skin abnormality seen?
  b What is its cause?

67 This thirty-eight year old woman has angina pectoris.
  a What abnormality is shown?
  b What is its significance here?

66

67

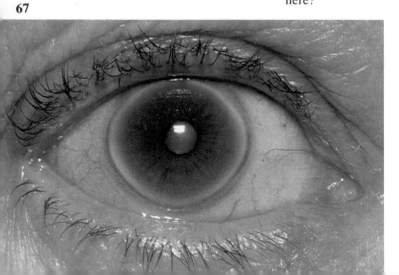

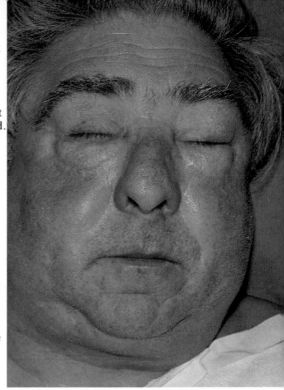

68 This patient became acutely dyspnoeic shortly after a diagnostic procedure was carried out on a general medical ward.
  a What name is given to the appearance seen here?
  b Which diagnostic procedure was performed?

69 This patient, who has recently developed a symmetrical polyarthropathy affecting hands and feet, now complains of altered sensation over both feet, and of a 'drop foot' on the left. The lesions shown here were preceded by painless reddish black spots in the same sites.
  a What are the lesions shown?
  b What is the likely underlying joint disorder?
  c What is the likely cause of her neurological symptoms?

69

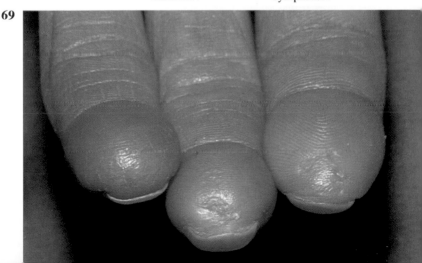

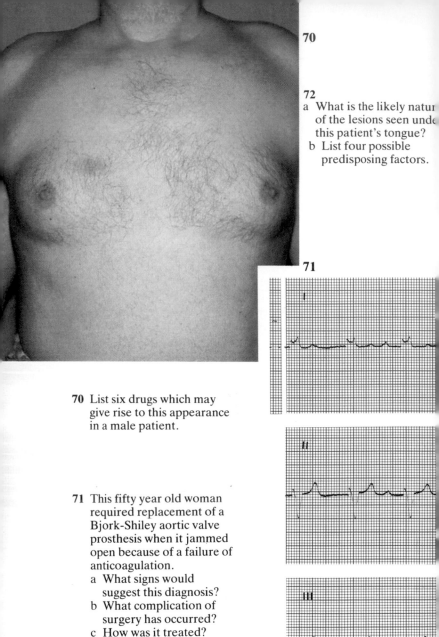

72
a What is the likely natur
of the lesions seen unde
this patient's tongue?
b List four possible
predisposing factors.

71

70 List six drugs which may
give rise to this appearance
in a male patient.

71 This fifty year old woman
required replacement of a
Bjork-Shiley aortic valve
prosthesis when it jammed
open because of a failure of
anticoagulation.
a What signs would
suggest this diagnosis?
b What complication of
surgery has occurred?
c How was it treated?

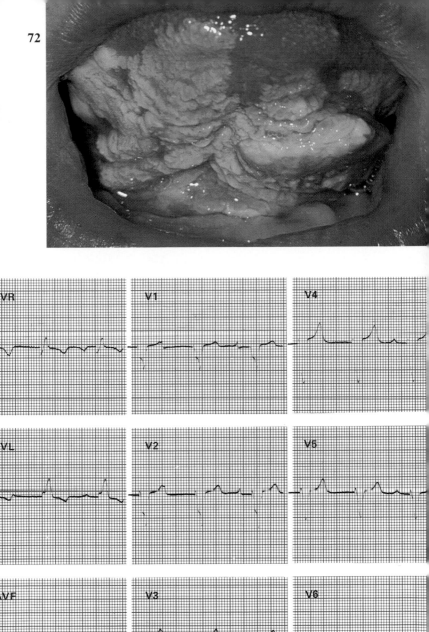

72

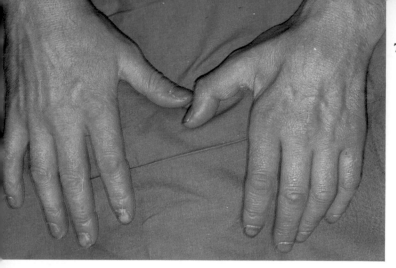

73 and 74 This patient has been referred for assessment of atypical angina pectoris.
  a What abnormality is seen in the hands?
  b What abnormalities are seen on chest x-ray?
  c What is the cause of his chest pain?

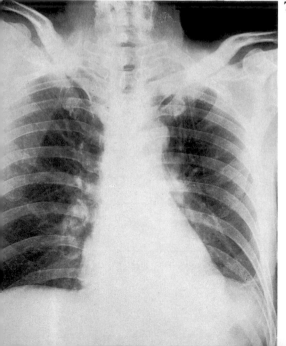

75

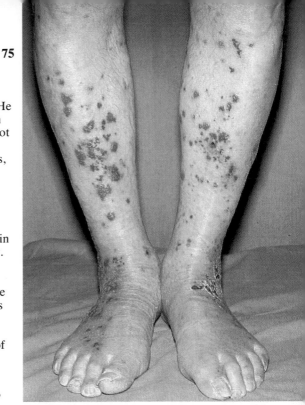

This seventy year old patient complains of altered sensation in the skin of his feet and legs. He has patchy sensory loss in both legs, weakness of foot eversion, ankle dorsiflexion on both sides, and of foot inversion on the left. His current medication includes hydralazine 25 mg twice daily. Urinalysis reveals traces of blood and protein but no other abnormality.

a What cutaneous abnormality is seen?

b What is the cause of the neurological symptoms and signs?

c What is the likely diagnosis in a patient of this age and sex?

d What blood test abnormalities would support this diagnosis?

76

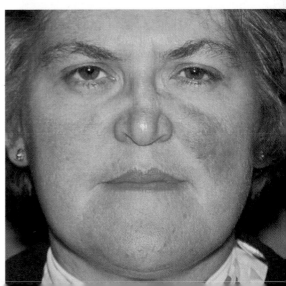

a What two abnormalities are visible on this patient's face?

b What are the two principal differential diagnoses?

c What simple bedside investigation may differentiate between the two?

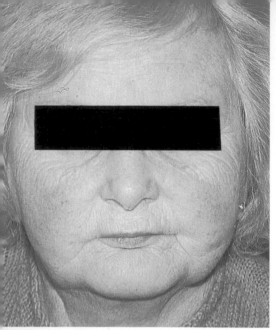

77 This patient is receiving thyroxine replacement therapy. She complains of cold intolerance.
   a Which physical sign best correlates with inadequate replacement?
   b Which single biochemical investigation is the most useful guide to adequacy of replacement in primary hypothyroidism?

77

78

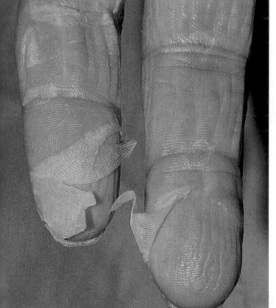

78 This abnormality developed two weeks after this patient had a sore throat.
   a Which infectious cause of sore throat is typically associated with this appearance?
   b What are the principal non-suppurative complications of this infection?

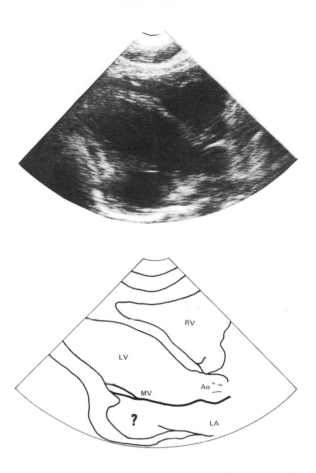

79 This cross-sectional echocardiogram is from a forty-five year old man who has an abnormal ECG. Following an episode of prolonged retrosternal and interscapular pain eight weeks ago, he has complained of exertional dyspnoea and orthopnoea.

   a What abnormality is seen on the echocardiogram (subcostal four-chamber view)?

   b What abnormalities may be present on his ECG?

   c Which cardiac murmur may be present?

        RV Right ventricle
        LV Left ventricle
        MV Mitral valve
        Ao Aorta
        LA Left atrium

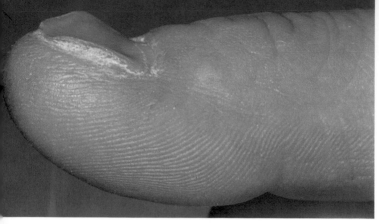

80

80 This patient complains of dysphagia.

    a What abnormality is shown?   b How may this relate to the complaint?

81

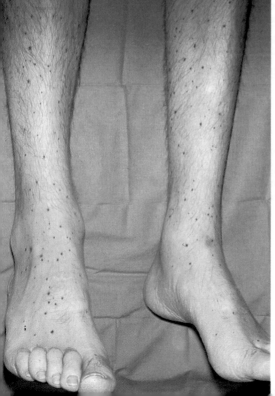

81

This patient's peripheral blood film is abnormal.

a What abnormality should be sought on abdominal examination?

b What diagnostic value would this abnormality have?

c If abdominal examination is normal, what is the likely finding on histology of bone marrow aspirate?

82

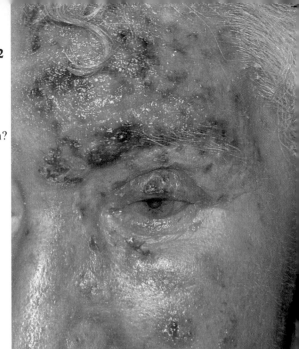

82 a What is this condition?
   b What are the
     complications of this
     condition?

83

a Describe the
  abnormalities shown in
  this optic fundus.
b State the underlying
  disorder.

83

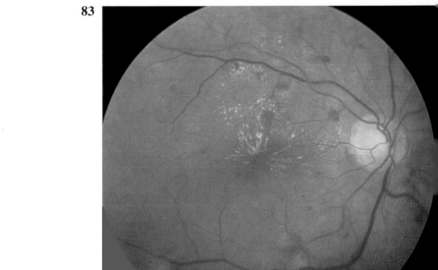

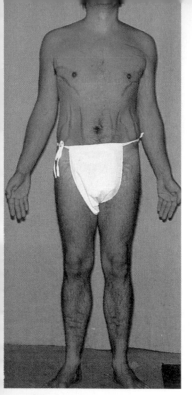

84

84 and 85 These patients are suffering from the same condition. They have undergone the same abdominal surgical operation.
  a What two abnormalities are seen in the male patient's skin?
  b What neurological abnormality does the female patient have?
  c What diagnosis is common to both?

85

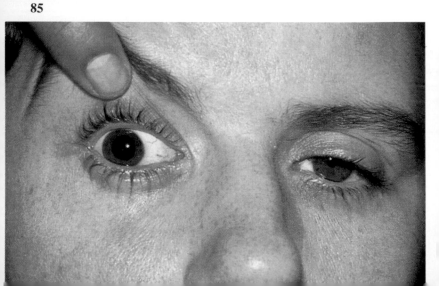

86 This man has chronic lymphocytic leukaemia.
  a What is the origin of the abnormal cell line?
  b What abnormalities of gamma globulins may be found in this disease?
  c What are the two major causes of anaemia in this disease?
  d What characteristic chromosomal abnormality is often present?

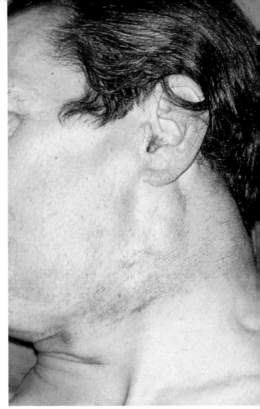

87 This patient has primary osteoarthrosis.
  a What names are given to the swellings seen in
  i) the distal interphalangeal joints?
  ii) the proximal interphalangeal joints?
  b What is the nature of the swelling?

86

87

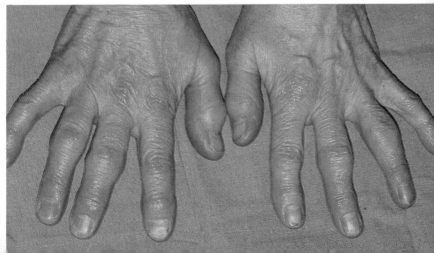

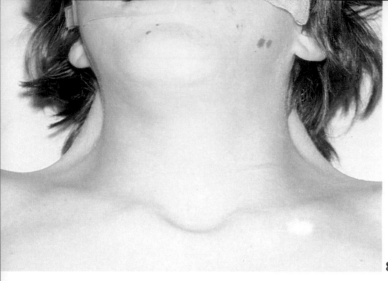

88

88 This patient has a congenital cardiovascular lesion.
   a What underlying problem is suggested by the appearance of her neck?
   b What clinical features of the cardiovascular lesion may be present?

89 Since a fall on outstretched hands three months ago this patient complains
   of persistent pain at the base of the thumb.
   What two abnormalities are seen in these x-rays?

89

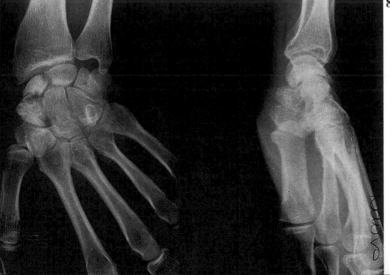

90 a Describe three
abnormalities present.
  b What is the diagnosis?

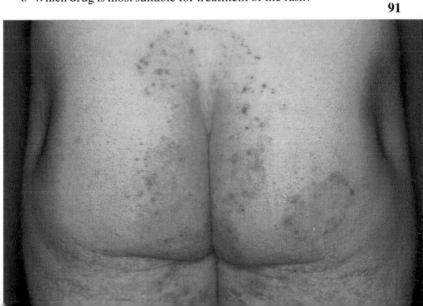

90

91 a What is the cause of this patient's itchy rash?
  b Which drug is most suitable for treatment of the rash?

91

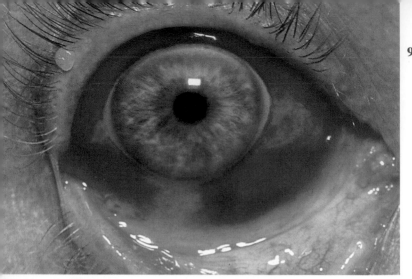

92

This thirty-nine year old man was knocked out in a road traffic accident. He was fully alert when seen initially but his conscious level deteriorated over the subsequent two hours. By the time of his arrival in hospital he had generalised increased muscle tone and bilateral extensor plantar responses.

a What diagnosis does his appearance suggest?

b What action is indicated?

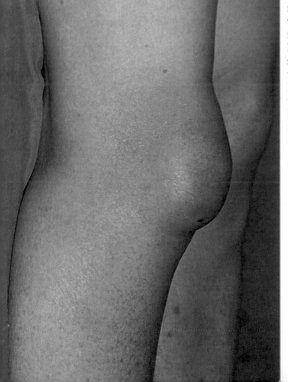

93 a What is this condition?

b Which organism is usually responsible?

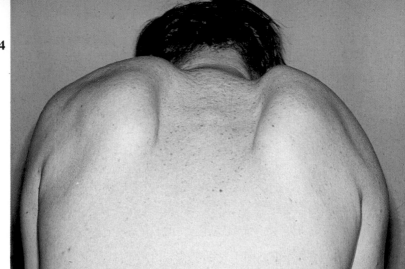

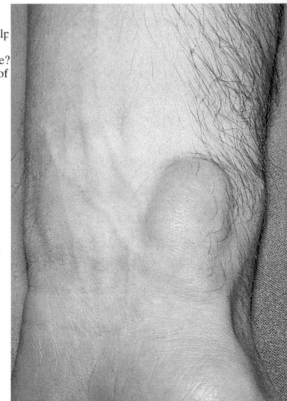

94 This patient has spinal muscular atrophy.
  a What features may help differentiate it from motor neurone disease?
  b What is the mainstay of treatment?

95 This man complains of a painless swelling on his wrist.
  a What is the likely diagnosis?
  b From what structure does it arise?
  c Is "text-book treatment" effective?

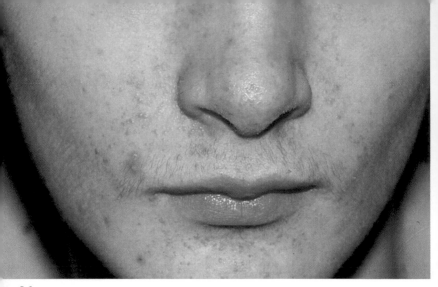

96

96 and 97 This patient has epilepsy. He is of average intelligence.
    a What underlying diagnosis is suggested by his facies? What name is given to the facial lesions?
    b What abnormalities are seen in the skin of his trunk?
    c What is the usual cause of epilepsy in this condition?
    d What two other skin abnormalities are typical of this disorder?

97

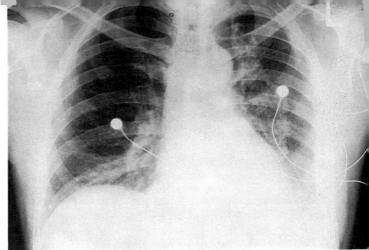

98 This x-ray was taken
during a routine medical
check up. The patient is
free of symptoms and has
no previous history of
acute respiratory or cardiac
illness.
  a What principal
    abnormality is seen on
    chest x-ray?
  b What is the most likely
    cause?
  c List three other
    respiratory
    complications of the
    underlying cause.

99 a What name is given to
    this rash?
  b What is the causative
    agent?
  c Does malignant
    transformation occur in
    these lesions?
  d What underlying
    medical disorder should
    be considered?

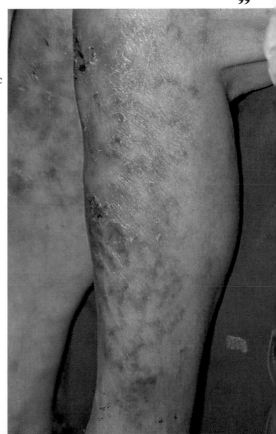

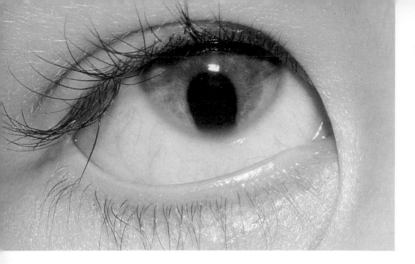

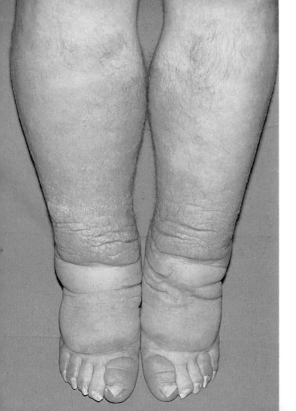

100

a What name is given to this abnormality?

b What is the cause?

c What is its significance?

101

a What is this?

b What is the underlying diagnosis?

c What treatment is available for the condition shown?

102

Following a Mediterranean holiday this patient was disappointed by his rather patchy suntan. Since the suntan has faded he is aware of patchy areas of increased pigmentation.

a What is the name given to this condition?

b What is the cause?

c How may the diagnosis be established?

103

This lady was admitted to hospital in a toxic, confused state.

a What abnormality is shown here?

b What is the causative agent?

c What is its significance in relation to her presenting complaint?

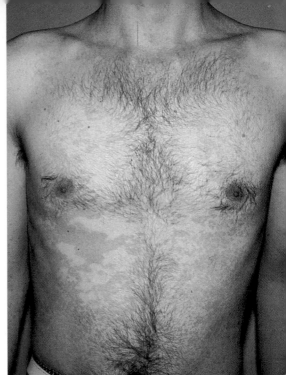

102

103

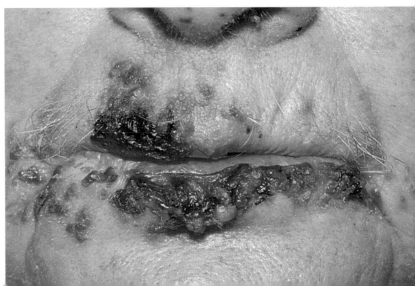

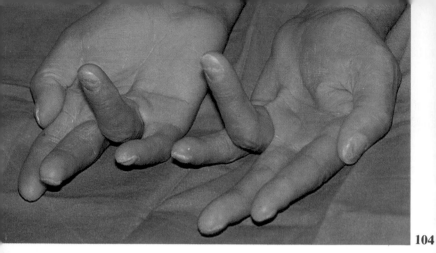

104

104 a A pattern of inheritance has been associated with this sign. What is it?
   b What neurological disorder has been associated with this sign?

105

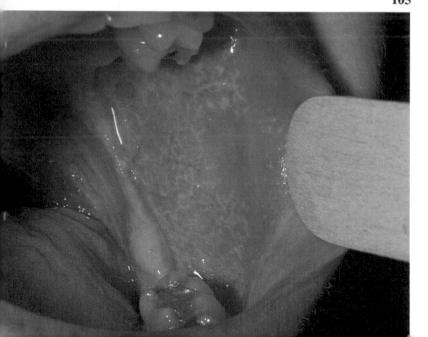

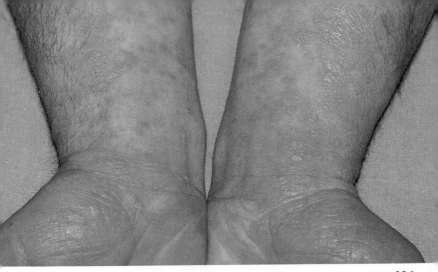

105 and 106 The itching eruption seen over this patient's wrists developed **106** over the course of two days.

  a How would you describe the skin lesions?

  b What is the most likely diagnosis?

  c What is the significance of buccal involvement in this condition?

107 This patient sustained a right-sided stroke two months ago.
Of what visual problem may he complain? **107**

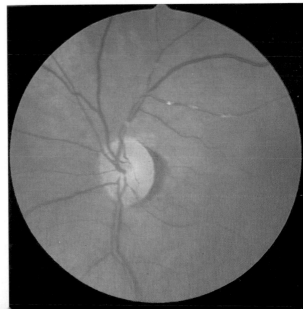

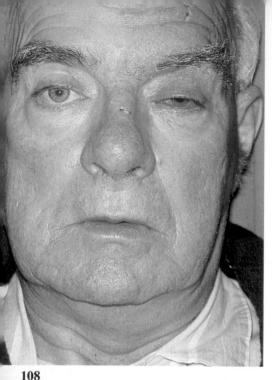

108 This man complained of pain above his left eye for several days before this appearance developed.

a What is the diagnosis?

b What is the significance of involvement of the nasociliary nerve in this disease?

c What therapies are useful?

109 This child's complaint of difficulty in rising from bed for some time was attributed to laziness.

a What abnormalities are seen in the chest x-ray?

b What is the most likely underlying diagnosis?

108

109

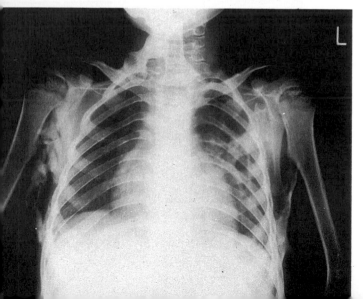

110

This patient complains of itchy spots around the ankle, which become swollen when rubbed. On a number of occasions she has experienced palpitations and lightheadedness shortly after scratching the ankle.

a What is the diagnosis?

b What histological abnormality is typical?

c What is the cause of her systemic symptoms?

d Which drugs should she avoid?

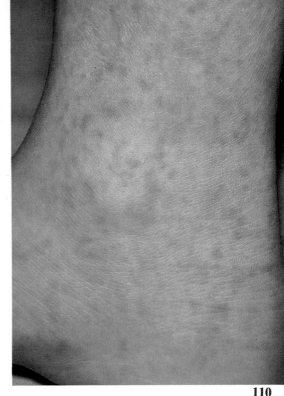

110

111 The lesion on this patient's forehead has increased rapidly in size over the past two to three weeks.

a What is the most likely diagnosis?

b What is the principal differential diagnosis?

111

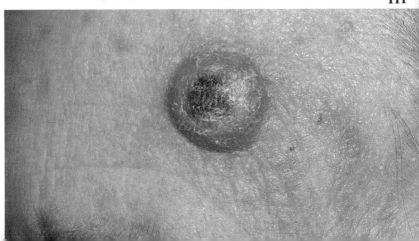

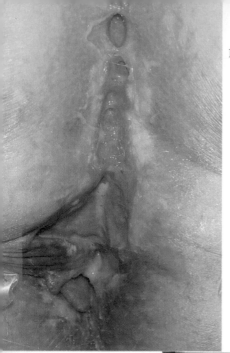

112 and 113 This patient has
a ten year history of
numerous surgical
procedures to large and
small bowel.
a What principal
abnormality is shown?
b What is the underlying
diagnosis?
c List four other
alimentary causes for
the skin lesions.

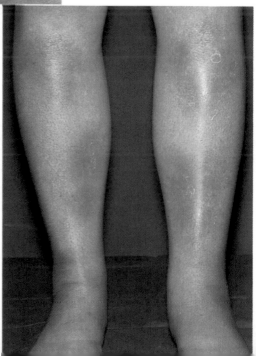

113

114
a What is likely to be this patient's principal complaint?
b What drug treatment is most likely to be helpful?

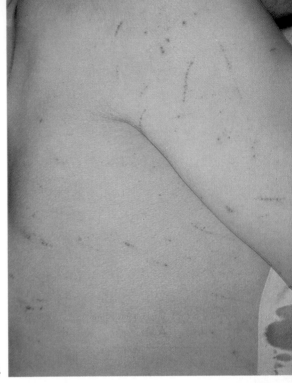

114

115

115
This seventy year old patient complains of gradually failing vision.
a What principal abnormality is seen in the optic fundus?
b What is the most likely cause of his visual deterioration?
c Which structure is primarily affected?

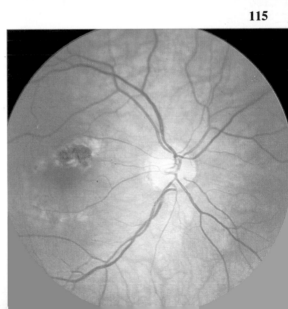

116

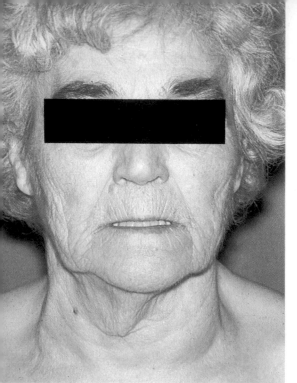

This patient with long-standing anaemia gives a two month history of weight loss and epigastric fullness after meals.
She has a left-sided ptosis

a What abnormality is seen in her neck?

b How does this relate to the eyelid abnormality?

c How might these relate to her presenting symptoms?

116

117 a What is this condition?

b What are the clinical features of this disorder?

117

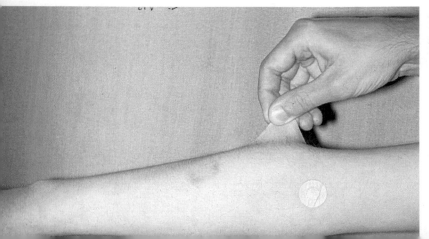

118

a What is the abnormality?

b What does it indicate?

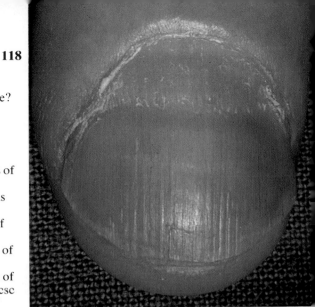

119

This patient complains of severe pain above the right knee joint and has recently lost weight.

a What abnormality of the shins is shown?

b What are the causes of this?

c Which complication of the commoner of these may have occurred?

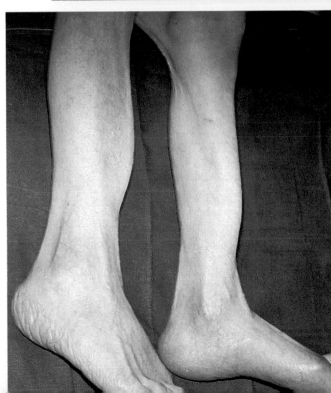

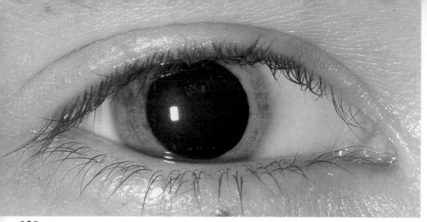

120

120 and 121 This child suffers from an unusual, inherited disorder
of mesenchymal tissue. He is tall for his age, with disproportionately
long extremities.
a What name is given to the abnormal appearance of the hands?
b What ocular abnormality is seen?
c What is the diagnosis and how is it usually inherited?
d Which disorder of metabolism may have similar clinical features?

121

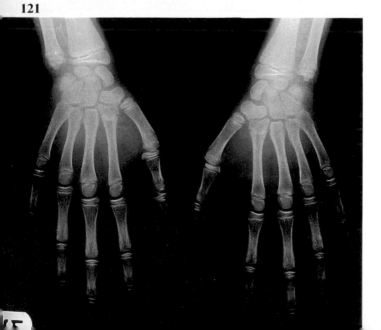

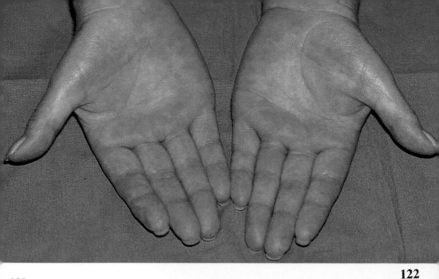

122
a What abnormality is seen in the skin of these hands?
b List five conditions which may be associated with these appearances.

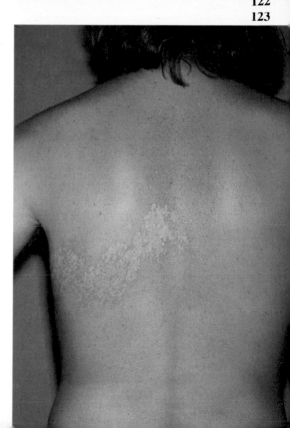

123
This young patient complains of recurrent lancinating pains under his left shoulder and anteriorly in his left lower chest.
What is the most likely cause?

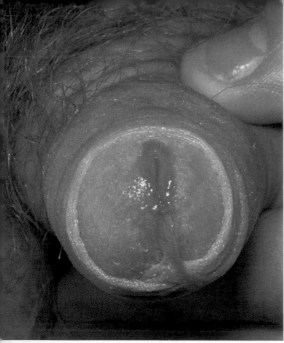

124

124 and 125 This patient
complains of dysuria and
of painful heels.
a What abnormalities are
seen on the x-ray?
b What is the most likely
diagnosis?

125

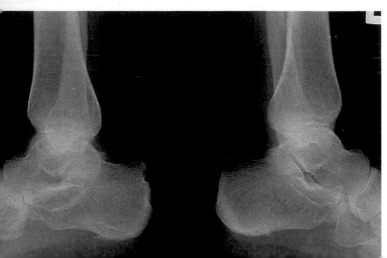

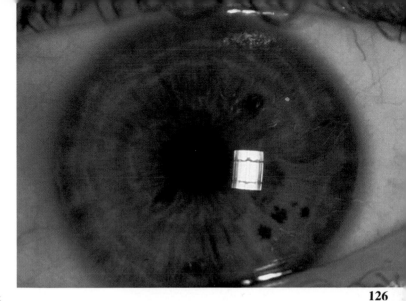

126

126
This patient has chronic renal failure.
a What is the abnormality?
b What surgical procedure may be necessary?

127
a Name two differential diagnoses of this neck swelling.
b How is the diagnosis established?

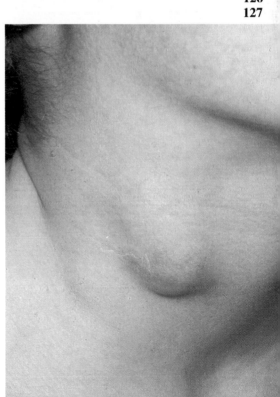

127

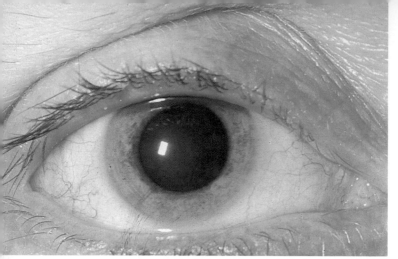

128

129

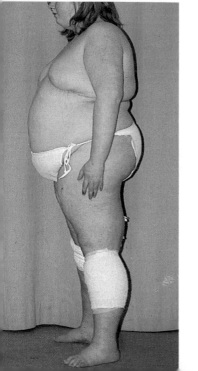

128 This forty-two year old
woman complains of
failing visual acuity.
  a What ocular
     abnormality is visible?
  b What is the most likely
     underlying cause?
  c List four other ocular
     features of this
     disorder.

129 This obese seventeen year
old girl has Prader-Willi
syndrome.
  a List four other features
     of this disease.
  b Name three other
     conditions which may
     have similar features.

130

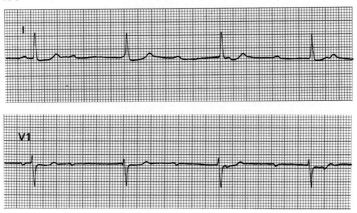

130 This asymptomatic thirty year old man was noted to have a bradycardia at an insurance medical. An ECG was performed.
a What rhythm is shown?
b What is the probable aetiology?
c Which further investigation would help establish the diagnosis?
d What treatment is indicated?

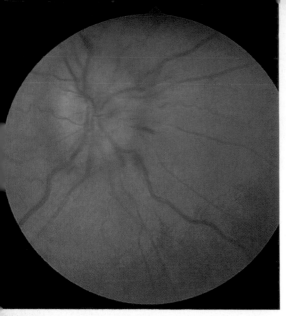

131

This is the fundus of a climber who complained of nausea, headache and unsteadiness after ascending 1,000m to 5,500m.

a What fundal abnormality is present?

b What is the diagnosis and which complication is developing?

c What treatment is indicated?

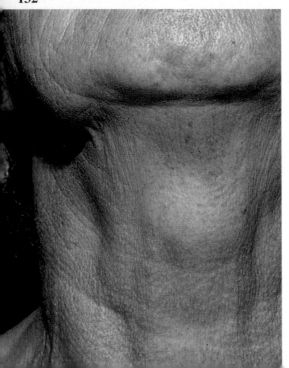

132

This swelling moves upward when the tongue is protruded.

a What is the diagnosis?

b From which pharyngeal pouch does it arise?

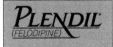

For hypertension,

These
calcium channel blockers
are dihydropyridines

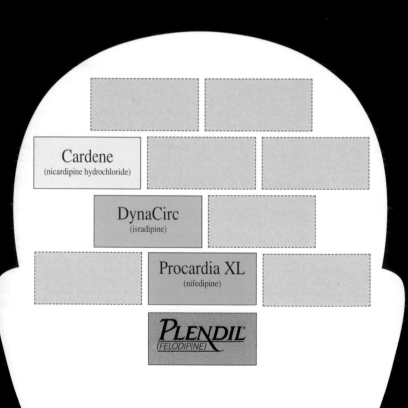

Only two dihydropyridine calcium channel blockers offer once-a-day dosing

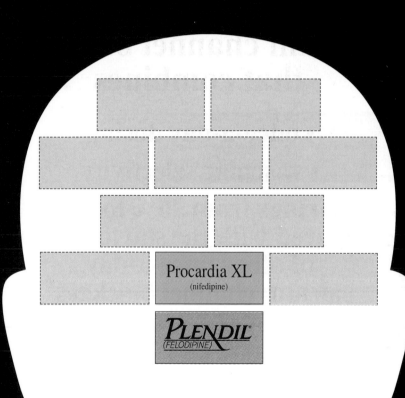

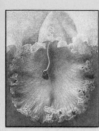
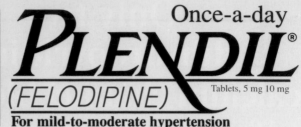

Once-a-day

PLENDIL®

Tablets, 5 mg 10 mg

(FELODIPINE)

For mild-to-moderate hypertension

A dihydropyridine calcium channel blocker that combines

- once-a-day dosing
- vascular selectivity
- savings from 26% to 59% compared with the starting doses of other once-a-day calcium channel blockers*

PLENDIL is contraindicated in patients who are hypersensitive to this product. Felodipine, like other calcium antagonists, may occasionally precipitate significant hypotension and, rarely, syncope. It may lead to reflex tachycardia, which in susceptible individuals may precipitate angina pectoris. (See ADVERSE REACTIONS.)

Although acute hemodynamic studies in a small number of patients with NYHA Class II or III heart failure treated with felodipine have not demonstrated negative inotropic effects, safety in patients with heart failure has not been established. Caution, therefore, should be exercised when using PLENDIL in patients with heart failure or compromised ventricular function, particularly in combination with a beta blocker.

*Based on the usual recommended starting dose(s) from the manufacturers' current product information for once-a-day calcium channel blockers for hypertension. Prices are manufacturers' direct prices, if available, or average wholesale prices from *MEDI-SPAN®* *Prescription Pricing Guide,* September 1992, based on the most frequently purchased package size for each strength.

Please see the Prescribing Information on the last pages of this book.

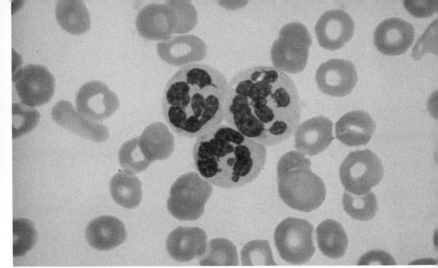

133 This is the blood film of a fifty year old woman who complained of poor balance, particularly in the dark, and tingling toes. Physical examination showed Rombergism, absent ankle and knee reflexes and extensor plantar responses.

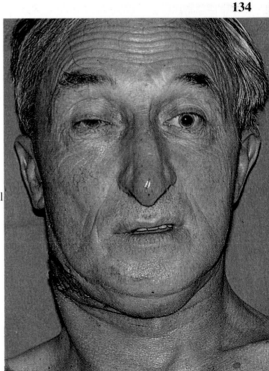

   a What two abnormalities are present in the blood film?

   b Which diagnosis is suggested by the film appearance and clinical description?

   c List three other neurological complications of this condition.

134 This taxi-driver was assaulted by his passenger.

   a What three abnormalities are present?

   b What is the diagnosis?

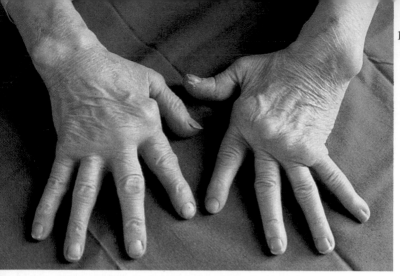

135

135 a List five abnormalities seen in these hands.
    b What is the likely diagnosis?
    c What principal complication is associated with the appearance of the distal ulna?

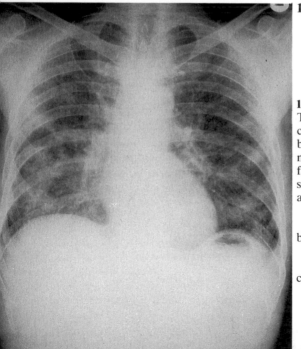

136

136
This pigeon breeder complains of cough and breathlessness of twelve months' duration. Bird fancier's lung is suspected.
a Describe the radiological abnormalities.
b Which investigations may help establish this diagnosis?
c List eight industrial forms of extrinsic allergic alveolitis.

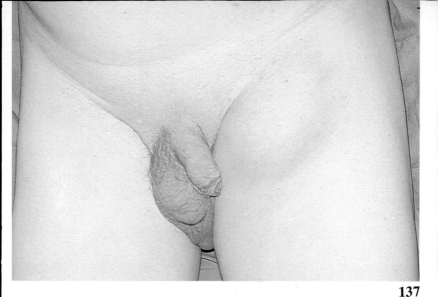

137 What is the differential diagnosis of the swelling in this six year old child's groin?

138 This sixty-four year old lady has chronic obstructive airways disease. Name the structures labelled 1 to 5 on the CT scan through the chest.

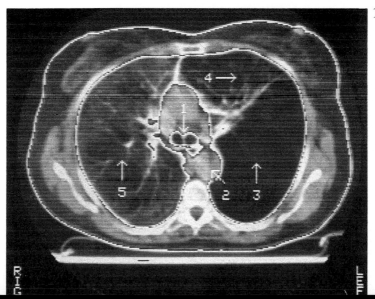

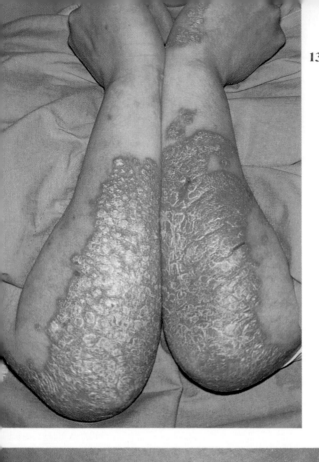

139

140

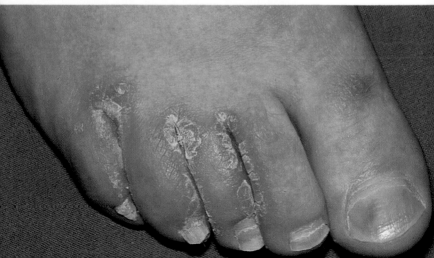

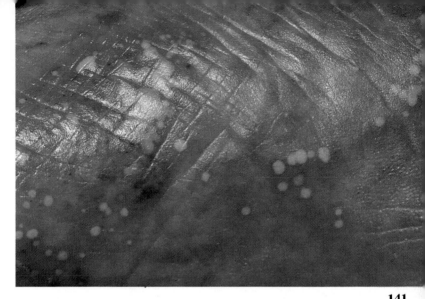

139, 140, 141 and 142 These patients all suffer from the same chronic skin disorder.
  a What skin disorder is this?
  b Name the morphological variety seen in each of these sites:
    i)   the forearms
    ii) the sole of the foot
    iii) the dorsum of the foot
    iv) the trunk.

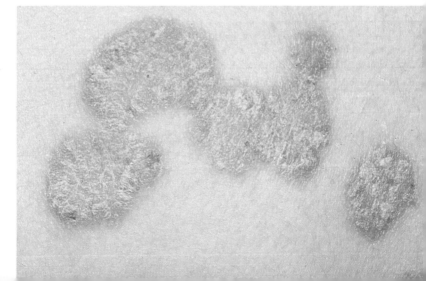

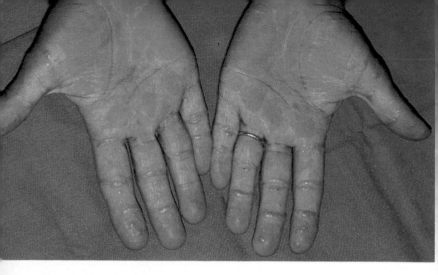

143 This forty year old woman complains of generalised pruritus and has noticed pale stools and dark urine for some months. She is mildly jaundiced.
  a What are the lesions seen in the skin creases on her fingers?
  b What is the likely diagnosis?
  c Which serological test is most useful in establishing the diagnosis?

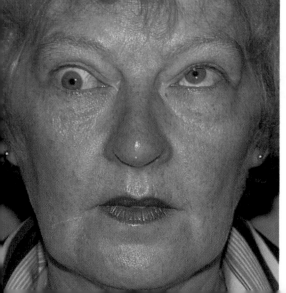

144

This patient is attempting to look upwards. Two years ago non-surgical treatment for an endocrine disorder was administered. Following this treatment the appearance of her eyes has worsened.
  a What is the diagnosis?
  b What treatment is she likely to have had?
  c What is likely to be her current endocrine status?

145

a What is the likely diagnosis?

b How may the diagnosis be confirmed?

c How should this disorder be treated?

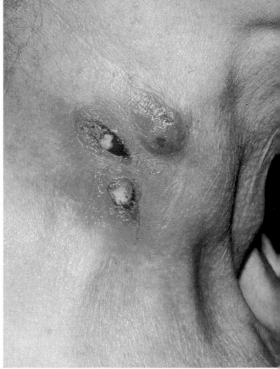

145

146

Since an attack of shingles several months ago (which produced a rash on his palate only), this patient has found difficulty with some movements of the left arm. He has been asked to shrug his shoulders.

a What two abnormalities can be seen?

b What is the neurological lesion?

146

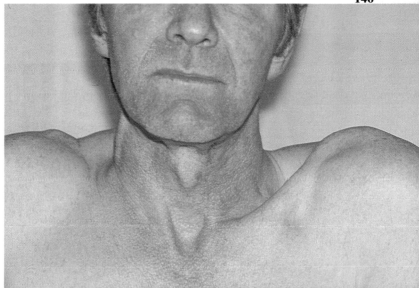

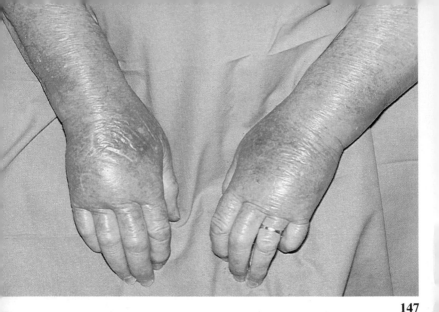

147

147 and 148 This woman has long history of productive cough. She recently complained of painful swollen wrists.
a What is the diagnosis?
b What may radiology of the hands and wrists show?
c Which other diseases are associated with the hand and wrist disorder?

148

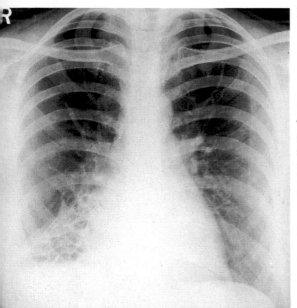

150
This child was referred for investigation of short stature and declining school performance. Bone age was retarded.
a What are the radiological abnormalities?
b What is the most likely diagnosis?
c Is growth hormone therapy indicated?

149

This man was admitted to hospital following a convulsion and was noted to have widespread bruising. Blood glucose was 2.3 mmol/l. A 5% glucose infusion was commenced. His platelet count was 140 x 10⁹/l, Hb 13.1 g/dl, MCV 110 fl. The blood film showed round macrocytosis and stomatocytosis. Prothrombin time was prolonged at 60 seconds. The following day he became confused and developed ocular paresis and nystagmus.

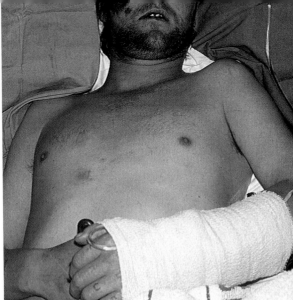

149

a What abnormality is present in addition to his bruising?

b What are the two likeliest causes of his convulsion? What is the probable underlying aetiology?

c How should the bleeding disorder be corrected?

d What is the cause of his deterioration and how could it have been prevented?

150

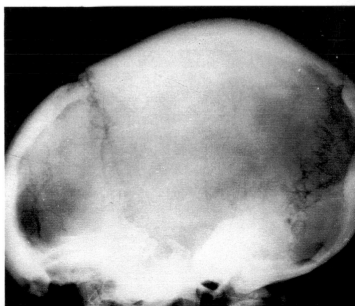

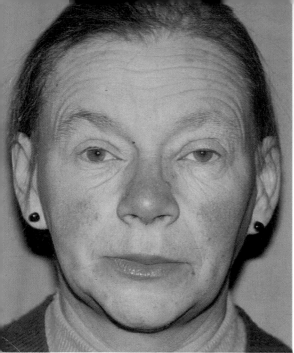

151

151
This patient complains of undue tiredness, dry skin and cold intolerance. Her skin appears to be becoming yellow.
a What is the diagnosis?
b Why is her skin becoming yellow?

152
This man has multiple myeloma. He complains of painful cold toes and fingers, especially in cold weather. His pedal pulses are normal.
a What is the likely cause of this appearance?
b What other cutaneous manifestations may occur?
c What therapy is available?
d What precautions should be taken when investigating this condition?

152

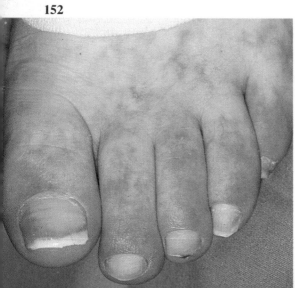

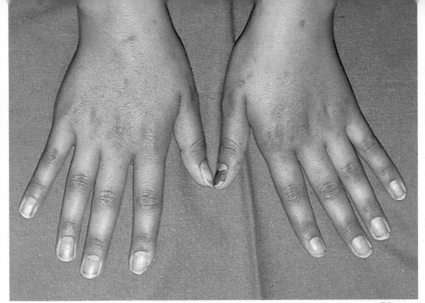

153

154

153 and 154
This patient
complains of tiredness.
a What principal
  abnormality is seen in
  i)   the hands?
  ii) the abdominal x-
       ray?
b What is the diagnosis,
  and what is the likely
  underlying cause in this
  case?

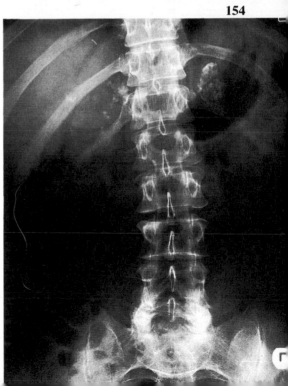

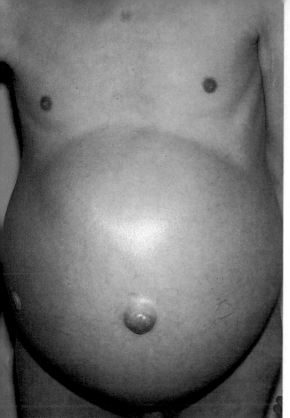

155
This patient with chronic compensated liver failure complained of increasingly painful abdominal distension and was admitted to hospital. A few days after admission he became mildly encephalopathic.

a What principal abnormality is seen here?

b What is likely to have precipitated his encephalopathy?

c List five other factors which may precipitate encephalopathy in these patients.

156
This man has multiple myeloma.

a What is this condition?

b Name three other disorders which may also predispose to this.

156

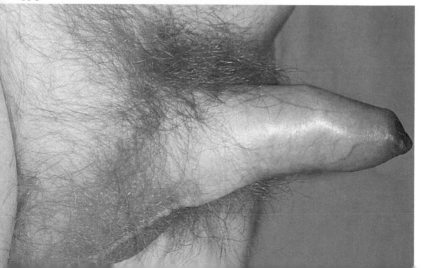

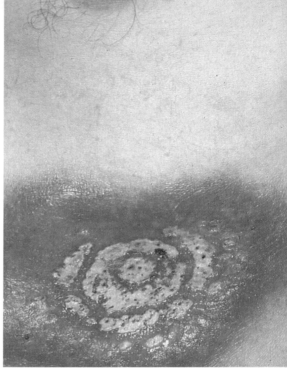

157 and 158
This patient
suffers from a chronic
gastrointestinal disorder.
He has had recurrent
scrotal lesions for years,
and over the past few
months has developed an
enlarging skin lesion on
the lower right chest wall.
a What name is given to
  the chest wall lesion?
b What is the underlying
  condition?

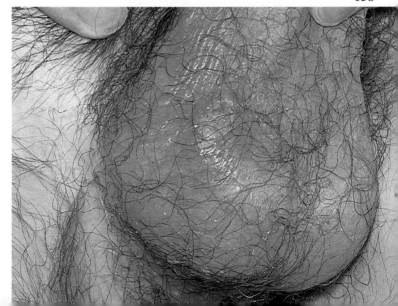

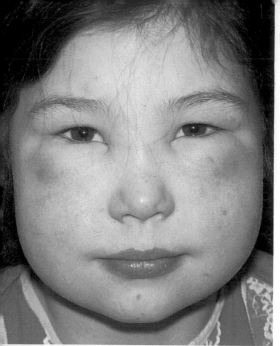

159
This young girl's serum calcium is low: she does not have clinical features of latent tetany.
a What is the clinical diagnosis?
b What is the most likely histological finding on biopsy of the appropriate organ?

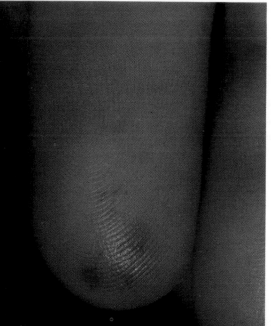

160

160
This patient presents with pyrexia.
a What eponymous abnormality is shown here?
b What is the likely diagnosis?
c What other clues to this condition may be found on clinical examination?

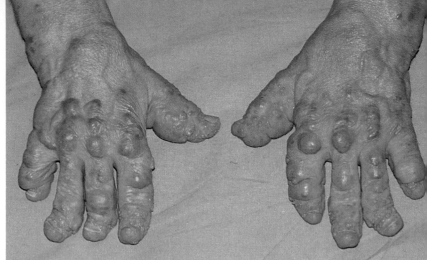

161
This patient complains of recurrent pain and swelling in all finger joints and both wrists.
What two main differential diagnoses are suggested?

162

a What description is given to the individual lesions shown?
b What is the diagnosis?
c Which two infectious diseases are most commonly recognised as precipitants?

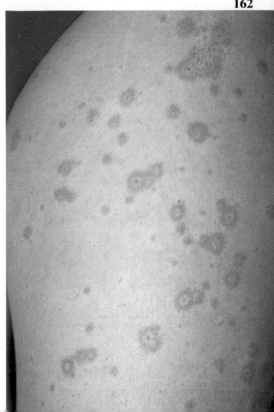

163

This woman is an insulin dependent diabetic.

a What is the diagnosis?

b Why is her pupil spared?

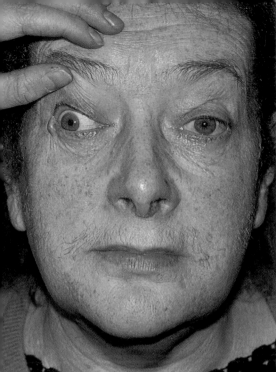

163

164 This patient feels as if she is walking 'on pebbles'.

a Of what condition is this foot deformity characteristic?

b What is the simplest means of relieving her symptoms?

164

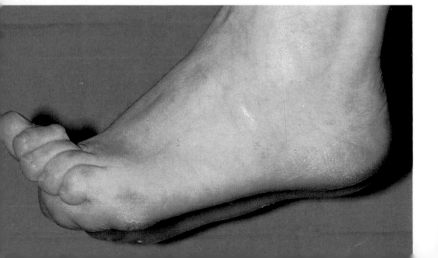

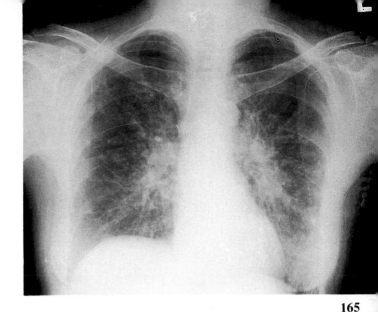

165 and 166 This patient complains of gradually progressive
exertional dyspnoea.
  a What abnormalities are seen in the chest film?
  b What abnormalities are seen in the hand x-rays?
  c What is the diagnosis?

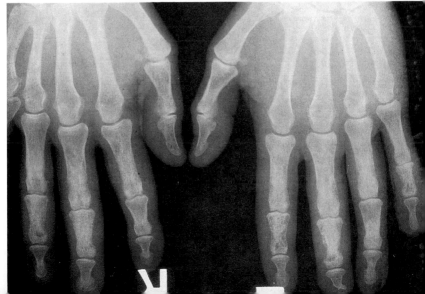

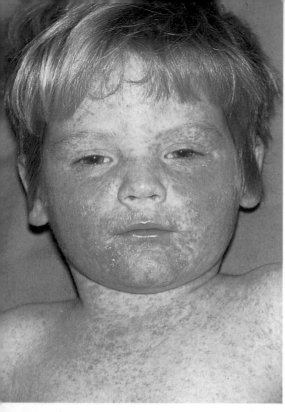

167 and 168
This boy
presented with right iliac
fossa pain. An
appendicectomy was
performed. He developed
this rash the following
day.
a What is the diagnosis?
b i)   What are the oral
        lesions and
   ii)   What is their
        significance?
c What may histology of
   the appendix show?

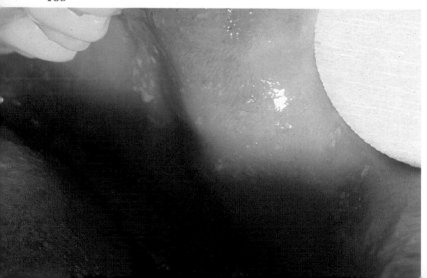

168

169

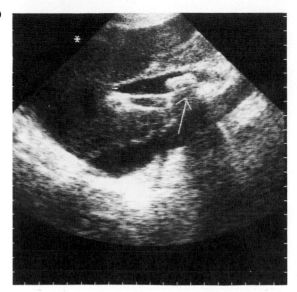

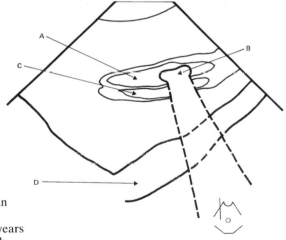

169
This fitty year old man who had a cholecystectomy six years ago now presents with jaundice, anorexia, nausea and vomiting.

a Name the features labelled 'A', 'B', 'C' and 'D' shown on this para-sagittal scan of the upper abdomen.

b List three other non-operative investigations which might be useful in demonstrating the biliary abnormality.

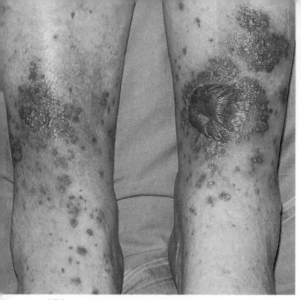

170

171

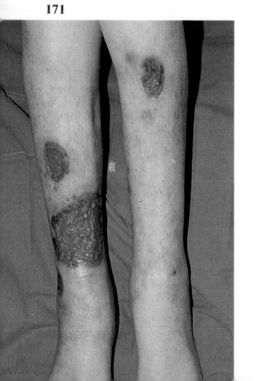

170 and 171 These patients both have rheumatoid arthritis.
a The lesions seen in both patients' lower legs have a common pathogenesis. What is it?
b List three other cutaneous manifestations of rheumatoid arthritis.

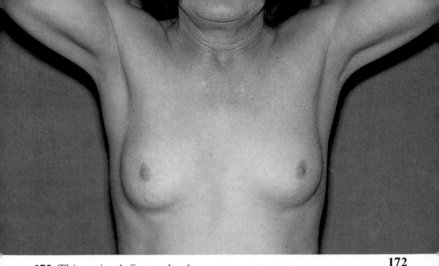

172 This patient's first and only pregnancy, twenty years ago, was
complicated by retained placenta and prolonged post-partum
haemorrhage.
  a What non-artefactual abnormality is seen here?
  b What is the likely diagnosis?
  c What are the usual early clinical features of this condition, following
     recovery from the precipitating illness?

173
This patient has a positive
serum Venereal Diseases
Research Laboratories
(VDRL) test.
a What abnormality is
   seen in his scalp?
b Suggest three possible
   diagnoses.

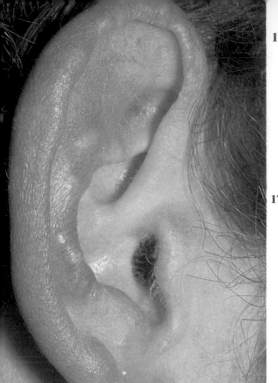

174

174 and 175 This patient has
groups of lesions, similar
to those seen on the ear
and hand, on his feet and
arms. He has no joint
symptoms, but complains
of recent weight loss and
polydipsia.
  a Of which non-infective
    skin condition are these
    appearances typical?
  b Which metabolic
    disorder may be
    associated with this
    condition?

175

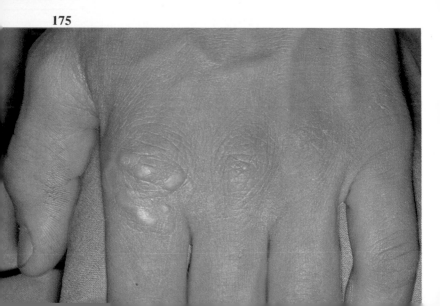

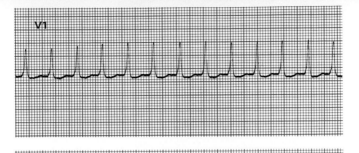

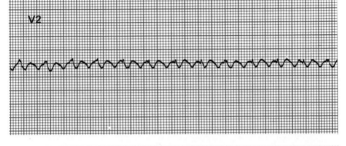

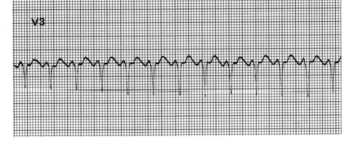

176 This man complained of palpitations and a tachycardia of 150 beats per minute was noted.

a What is the dysrhythmia?

b What auscultatory finding may help differentiate this from paroxysmal atrial tachycardia?

c What are the effects of digoxin administration on this dysrhythmia?

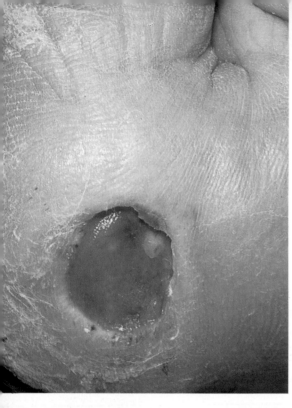

177

177 and 178

a What abnormalities are shown on this patient's foot and foot x-ray?

b What is the most likely diagnosis?

c Which organisms may be responsible?

178

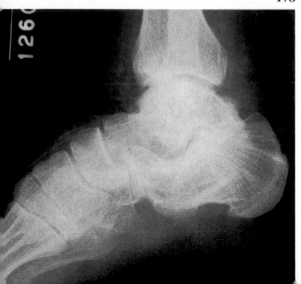

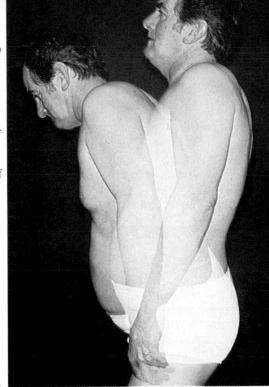

179 This fifty-eight year old patient complains of back pain and stiffness, especially after periods of rest, of six months duration. The picture illustrates his full range of spinal flexion and extension. The distance from the sacrum to the twelfth dorsal vertebra varies four centimetres during this exercise. What is the most likely diagnosis?

180

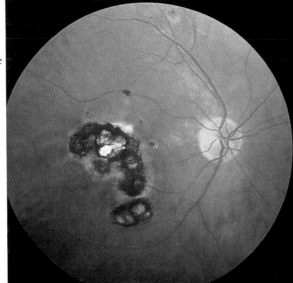

180
This woman has defective vision because of a lesion present since birth.
a What abnormality of vision is likely?
b What is the underlying cause?
c Will her younger sister suffer from the same condition?

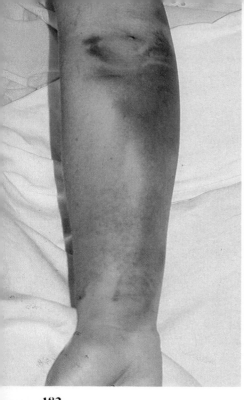

181 and 182 This patient complained of lethargy, pallor and increased bruising. She was noted to bleed excessively from venepuncture sites. Her haemoglobin was 8 g/dl, white cell count 178 x 10⁹/1 and platelet count 21 x 10⁹/1. Prothrombin time and partial thromboplastin time were prolonged, fibrinogen reduced, and fibrin degradation products present in excess.
a What underlying diagnosis does this blood film suggest?
b Which complication has occurred?

182

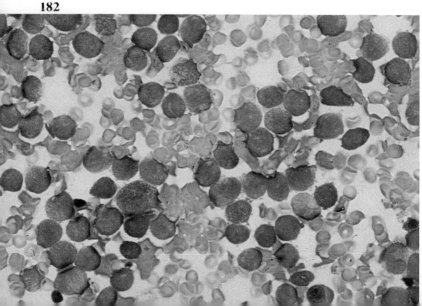

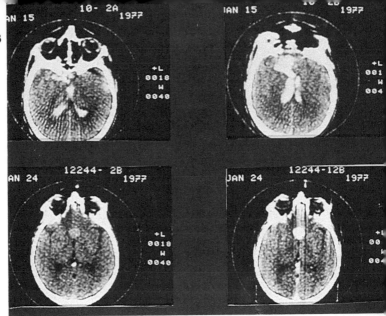

183

183 a What abnormalities does this cerebral CT scan show?

b What is the probable diagnosis?

184

184
This child was thought to be deaf by his parents. This appearance was present bilaterally.

a Describe the appearance and suggest the likely diagnosis.

b What abnormality should be detectable on testing hearing with a tuning fork?

c Are antibiotics indicated for this condition?

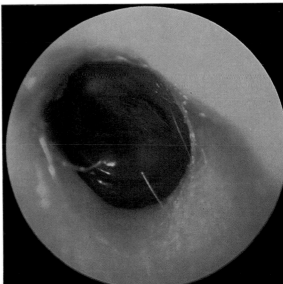

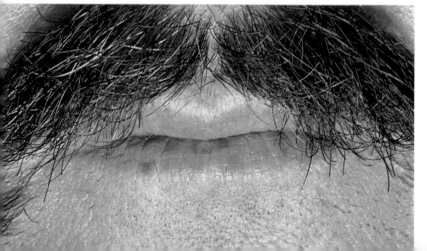

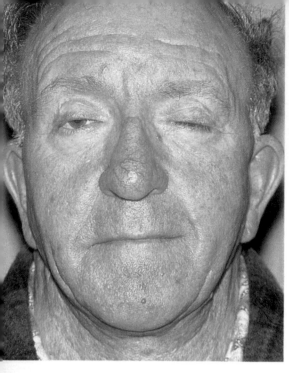

185

185
This sixty-two year old gardener has been unable to work because of increasing weakness, which progresses throughout the day. He has recently experienced several transient episodes of diplopia and of regurgitation of fluids down his nose.
a What ocular abnormality is shown?
b What is the likely diagnosis?
c How can this be confirmed simply?
d Is this age of onset unusual?

186 a What abnormality of the lips is shown?
   b With what is this associated and what is the disease called?
   c Is this condition associated with malignancy?

186

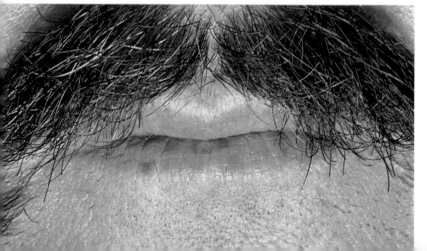

187

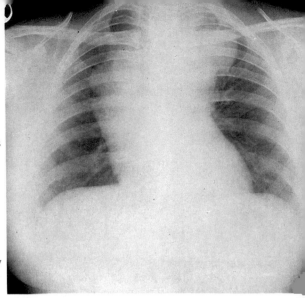

187

This thirty-two year old female patient complains of generalised pruritus. Examination reveals no dermatological abnormality.

a What abnormality is seen on chest x-ray?

b What is the likely diagnosis?

c What is the most likely histological variety in this case?

188

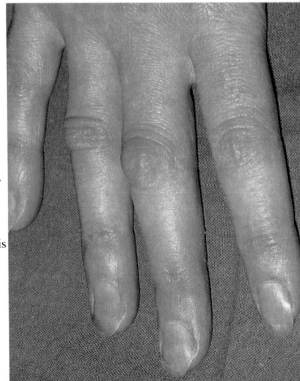

188

This woman complained about the unsightly appearance of her hands.

a What abnormality is present?

b How is the condition acquired?

c With which condition is this associated?

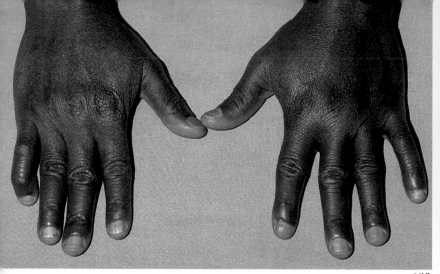

189 and 190 These two patients are suffering from the same condition. The first complains of intense pain in the left hand of two days duration. The second (whose hand x-ray is shown) has no symptoms.
- a What principal abnormality is seen
  - i) in the hands?
  - ii) in the x-rays?
- b What is the most likely diagnosis, and what is the causative agent?
- c What is the geographical distribution of this disorder?

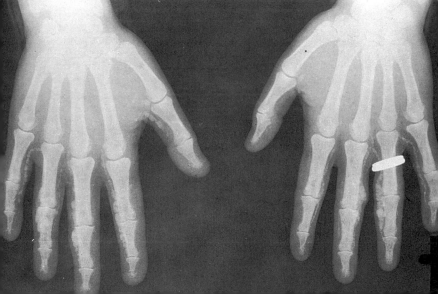

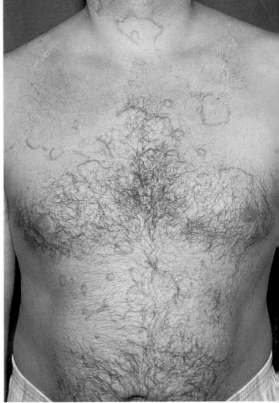

191

This patient was admitted
to hospital after a major
gastrointestinal bleed.
The morning after
admission this skin rash
was seen to have
developed. There is no
history of similar rashes.
a What type of rash is
    this?
b Suggest two possible
    causes.

192

a What name is given to
    the ocular abnormality
    seen?
b Suggest two possible
    causes.

192

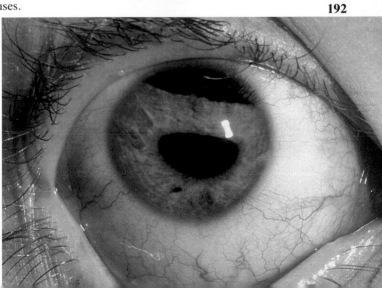

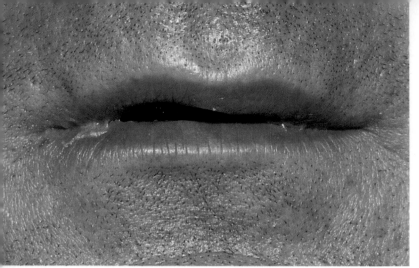

193

193 This man was seen two hours after swallowing a quantity of weed killer. His appearance did not change with oxygen administration.

a What abnormality is present and what is the likely cause?
b What type of weedkiller has he taken?
c What immediate treatment should be given?

194

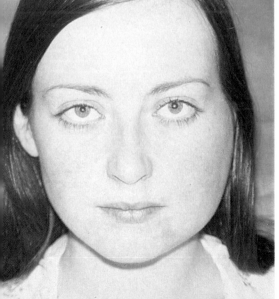

194

This patient was admitted to hospital complaining of headache, neck stiffness, and drowsiness. The following day this facial appearance had developed.

a What is the likely diagnosis?
b What would lumbar puncture show?
c How is the diagnosis confirmed?

ANSWERS

The answers given below are necessarily brief as the aim of the series is to stimulate self-learning through further reading.

1 a A polypoid vascular tumour is invading the middle ear.
  b Glomus jugulare with involvement of the IXth, Xth and XIth cranial nerves.
  c Radiotherapy is often required when the tumour has caused extensive local destruction, but smaller tumours may be treated surgically.

2 a Leishman-Donovan bodies in a monocyte; visceral leishmaniasis.
  b Phlebotomus sandflies.
  c Pentavalent antimonials such as sodium stilbogluconate.

3 Rupture of the supraspinatus tendon.

4 a Prepatellar bursitis.
  b Housemaid's knee.
  c No. The prepatellar bursa does not communicate with the knee joint.

5 a Temporal (cranial, giant cell) arteritis. The symptoms are, however, not specific for this disorder.
  b i) Lingual and jaw claudication.
    ii) Raynaud's phenomenon of the tongue.
  c None. Tortuosity of the extracranial arteries is a normal finding at this age.

6 a Pressure sores.
  b Secondary amyloidosis, with renal glomerular involvement.
  c Rectal biopsy.

7 and 8
  a 'Rockerbottom' foot.
  b Trisomy 18. Edwards' syndrome.
  c Poor. Few children survive into their second year.
    (Average male survival is under sixty days. Females tend to survive longer).

9 a These represent pericardial fluid.
  b i) Variable opening of the mitral valve.
    ii) Early collapse in systole of the right ventricular outflow tract.
       These are signs of cardiac tamponade.
  c Pericardiocentesis. This is a relatively simple procedure under ultrasonic control.

10 a Strawberry naevus (angiomatous naevus, cavernous naevus/ haemangioma).
  b i)   Failure to resolve spontaneously (cosmetic).
    ii) Ulceration.
    iii) Feeding difficulty.
    iv) Haemorrhage.

11 a Herpetic whitlows.
  b Electron microscopy of aspirated blister fluid.

12 a Ichthyosis.
  b Hodgkin's disease.
  c i)   Other malignancies — lymphosarcoma, mycosis fungoides, Kaposi's sarcoma.
    ii) Leprosy.
    iii) Malnutrition — especially vitamin A deficiency.

13 a Argyll Robertson pupil
  b False.
    The Argyll Robertson pupil of neurosyphilis is characteristically small. A dilated pupil which reacts as described may be found in association with pineal tumours, diabetes mellitus and brainstem encephalitis.

14 a Hypermetropia.
  b Pseudopapilloedema (may be a normal feature of the hypermetropic fundus).

15 a Aplastic anaemia.
  b Absence of lymphadenopathy or hepatosplenomegaly which would suggest an alternative cause of pancytopaenia.
  c The marrow is hypoplastic with extensive fatty replacement.
  d Sulphamethoxazole.

16, 17 and 18
  a Multiple discrete lytic lesions in the skull. Lytic lesions of the lumbar vertebral bodies. Compression fracture of the body of the twelfth thoracic vertebral body.
  b Hyperviscosity syndrome due to polymerisation of the excessive immunoglobulin and/or thrombocytopaenia and anaemia due to marrow failure.
  c Serum creatinine, blood urea, haemoglobin, and serum albumin.

19 and 20
  a i)   Left Horner's syndrome.
    ii) Wasting of first dorsal interosseus muscle on both sides; multiple healed scars, mostly of the right hand, claw hand on the right.
  b i)   Syringomyelia.
    ii) Intrinsic tumour of the cervical spinal cord (eg ependymoma, glioma).
         Bilateral lower brachial plexus lesions (eg in association with Pancoast tumours) unlikely.

21 a Proptosis (this patient may also have exophthalmos — sclera visible between the iris and lower lid — but this is best seen from the front).

 b Exophthalmometer — measuring the distance between the lateral angle of the orbit and an imaginary line perpendicular to the cornea's anterior surface.

22 a i) Striae (old).
 ii) Widening of the primary areola.
 iii) Montgomery's tubercles.
 iv) Dilated superficial veins.

 b Pregnancy.

 c Between eight and twelve weeks ago. (Darkening of the primary areola, and development of the secondary areola, which occur from twelve and sixteen weeks onwards respectively, are not yet seen).

23 and 24

Hyperuricaemia — the first patient has tophaceous gout, the second patient has psoriasis.
(Severe exfoliative psoriasis with rapid epidermal cell division may lead to hyperuricaemia due to increased turnover of purines).

25 a Sinus tachycardia; P mitrale; anteroseptal myocardial infarction; ST elevation in leads V1 — 4.

 b He has developed a ventricular aneurysm. The P mitrale may indicate mitral regurgitation and dilatation of the left atrium.

 c A diffuse, often laterally displaced apex beat with a double or paradoxical impulse is characteristic of ventricular aneurysm; the murmur of mitral regurgitation may be present.

26 and 27

 a i) Irregular grey-brown discolouration.
 ii) Expansion of the lower end of the femur. (The Ehrlenmayer flask deformity).

 b Gaucher's disease.

 c Massive splenomegaly, hepatomegaly.

 d Raised serum acid phosphatase (of bony origin).

28 a Swelling over front and left lateral aspect of neck.

 b i) Isotopic thyroid scan.
 ii) Ultrasonic scan of thyroid.
 iii) Fine needle — aspiration biopsy.
 iv) (Serum thyroxine and tri-iodothyronine levels).
 v) (Serum thyroid antibodies).

 c i) Colloid cyst of thyroid.
 ii) Thyroid adenoma.
 iii) Thyroid carcinoma.

29 a He has developed an inhibitor to factor VIII.

 b Haemophiliac or von Willebrand patients transfused with factor VIII; post partum women; autoimmune diseases (e.g. systemic lupus erythematosus); drug reactions.

30 a Rheumatoid nodules.

    b Extensor aspect forearm, olecranon (as shown), sacrum, achilles tendon, extensor and flexor tendons in the hand; sclerae, myocardium, lung.

    c The presence of nodules is typically associated with seropositive and more aggressive rheumatoid arthritis.

31 a Malignant melanomata.

    b   i)   Surgery — wide excision + split skin grafting (from the unaffected limb) + (where practical) dissection of draining nodes.

         ii)   Chemotherapy
             — systemic: single (eg. Dacarbazine) or combined regimes.
             — regional perfusion (eg. phenylalanine mustard).

         iii) Radiotherapy (especially for malignant change in Hutchinson's lentigo).

         iv) Immunotherapy — BCG,
                                Vaccinia, corynebacterium parvum.

         v)   Hyperthermia.

32 a Short stature; infantile proportions — i.e. in ratio of trunk to limb; coarse facial features.

    b Juvenile hypothyroidism.

    c Measurement of serum thyroxine and thyroid stimulating hormone concentrations.

33 a Psoriasis.

    b Nail changes include   i) pitting
                           ii) onycholysis
                          iii) discoloration
                          iv) thickening.

34 and 35

    a No, intelligence is not affected.

    b The reflexes are often impaired with the exception of the ankle jerks.

    c No. It should be normal.

36 a Basal cell carcinoma (rodent ulcer). Squamous carcinoma is much less likely.

    b Conjunctival keratinisation and chronic keratitis. Inadequate radiation may induce metaplasia to squamous carcinoma.

    c i)   Surgical excision.
        ii) Cryotherapy.
        iii) Topical cytotoxic drugs such as 5-fluorouracil.

37 a The ulnar nerve.

    b There is wasting of the thenar eminence.

    c Either the ulnar nerve is supplying all the intrinsic muscles of the hand as it does in 2-3% of the population or the lesion is in the brachial plexus damaging the lower trunk.

38 Hydrochlorothiazide, chlorpropamide. (This is a photosensitive eruption).

39 a Lacework expansion of the marrow cavities with loss of the normal fine medullary trabeculation particularly in the phalanges.
   b Thalassaemia major.
   c Splenectomy (following which the peripheral platelet, white cell and nucleated red cell counts rise).
   d Pneumococcal infection.

40 a Sebaceous naevus.
   b Malignant transformation may occur (eg. basal cell carcinoma in approximately 20%).

41 a Brushfield's spots, around the iris.
   b Down's syndrome (trisomy 21).

42 a Looser's zones (pseudo fractures).
   b Osteomalacia.
   c Osteomalacia is well-recognised association of treatment with
      i)   Phenytoin.
      ii) Phenobarbitone.
      iii) Primidone.
      iv) Other enzyme inducer drugs.
      (Limited exposure to sunlight may contribute).

43 a Sunlight — these are solar keratoses.
   b These may be premalignant — Squamous carcinoma may develop.

44 Artefact
   (These are 'pinch' skin graft donor sites).

45 a Pyogenic granuloma.
   b Capillary proliferation.

46 and 47
   a Increased anteroposterior diameter ('barrel' chest)
   b Atopic eczema (which more typically affects the flexures).
   c i)   Conjunctivitis.
      ii) Atopic cataract.
      iii) Keratoconus (conical cornea).

48 a 'Hair on end' appearance.
   b Extramedullary haemopoiesis/expanded marrow cavity.
   c Thalassaemia major.

49 a Tinea incognito.
   b Steroid-modified ringworm infection.

50 a Ambiguous external genitalia with clitoromegaly and fusion of the labia.

    b Congenital adrenal hyperplasia of the salt-losing type.
    c 21-hydroxylase deficiency.

51 a Ascites, hepatomegaly and, less commonly, splenomegaly.
    b Pulsus paradoxus.
    c The jugular venous pressure is characteristically raised and rises further
       on inspiration (Kussmaul's sign).
    d Excision of the pericardium is the treatment of choice, in addition to
       the standard treatment of congestive cardiac failure.

52 and 53
    a i)   Swelling and erythema suggesting acute arthritis.
       ii) Erythematous, scaling, pustular eruption.
    b Gonococcal arthritis and dermatitis; anorectal gonorrhoea is the likely
       site of infection.
    c Culture of urine, blood, synovial fluid, rectal and urethral; smears and
       skin lesions.

54 a 1 in 4 (Autosomal dominant inheritance).
    b At present there is no reliable method of detecting Huntington's
       chorea prior to the onset of symptoms.
    c None. (Although cholestatic hepatitis associated with phenothiazine
       therapy may occur).

55 a Multiple shallow aphthous ulcers on reddened bases on the tongue, and
       several vesicles (pustules) on the thumb.
    b Primary herpes simplex — acute herpetic gingivostomatitis and
       herpetic whitlows.
    c Thumb-sucking.

56 a Hepatic bruit.
    b Hepatocellular carcinoma.
    c i)   Cirrhosis (especially haemochromatosis, can occur in any type).
       ii) Hepatitis B infection.
       iii) Aflatoxin (produced by aspergillus flavus).
       iv) Oral contraceptive (very rarely).

57 a Adult coeliac disease (gluten-sensitive enteropathy).
    b i)   Iron deficiency, secondary to malabsorption.
       ii) Hyposplenism — splenic atrophy.
    c i)   Small bowel lymphoma.
       ii) Ulcerative jejunoileitis.

58 a Achondroplasia.
    b Endochondral ossification.
    c Increasing paternal age.

59 a Bilateral hilar and mediastinal lymphadenopathy.
    b The linear lucency separating hilar from mediastinal nodes indicates
       that the nodes are discrete, and therefore more likely to be benign.

60 and 61
  a Gouty tophi.
  b Central nervous system.
  c i) Uric acid nephrolithiasis.
    ii) Uric acid nephropathy.
    iii) Hypertensive renal disease.

62 a i) 'Hound dog' facial expression.
    ii) Masseter, temporalis and sternomastoid wasting.
    iii) Frontal balding.
  b Myotonic dystrophy.

63 a Osgood Schlatter's disease.
    (Osteochondritis of the tibial tuberosity.)

64 a Increased pigmentation and presence of buccal pigmentation.
  b Adrenal insufficiency.
  c i) Plasma cortisol and response to tetracosactrin — low cortisol and diminished response.
    ii) Plasma adrenocorticotrophic hormone — greatly elevated.
  d i) Autoimmune disease of adrenal gland.
    ii) Tuberculosis.
    iii) Metastatic carcinoma.
    iv) Adrenalectomy.
    v) Systemic fungal infections.
    vi) Amyloidosis.

65 Adenocarcinoma (especially gastric). The illustration shows axillary acanthosis nigricans.

66 a Erythema ab igne.
  b Prolonged application of heat (via hot water bottle, poultices) for pain relief.

67 a Corneal arcus.
  b It suggests underlying hypercholesterolaemia; a potentially treatable risk factor in ischaemic heart disease.

68 a Surgical emphysema (note the dressing of a left upper intercostal drain).
  b Pleural aspiration/biopsy.

69 a Healed digital infarcts.
  b Rheumatoid arthritis.
  c Mononeuritis multiplex.
    (Early peripheral neuropathy is possible; secondary to vasculitic involvement of vasa nervorum).

70 i) Spironolactone.
    ii) Digitalis (possibly, digoxin).

iii) Oestrogens eg. stilboestrol.
iv) Isoniazid.
v) Ethionamide.
vi) Griseofulvin.
vii) Testosterone.
viii) Cimetidine.

71 a Loss of the prosthetic valve sounds and the development of the murmur of aortic regurgitation.
    b Complete heart block due to damage to the conducting system during valve replacement.
    c A permanent transvenous ventricular pacemaker was inserted.

72 a Leukoplakia. Intraepithelial/squamous carcinoma must be excluded by histology.
    b i) Tobacco smoking.
       ii) Local irritation — ill fitting dentures, dental caries.
       iii) Candida albicans infection.
       iv) Severe iron deficiency anaemia.

73 and 74

a Wasting of the small hand muscles (most noticeably 1st dorsal interosseus) on left.
b i) Opacity left apex.
   ii) Destruction of proximal end of 2nd left rib.
c Apical bronchogenic carcinoma (Pancoast tumour), with intercostal and brachial plexus nerve invasion.

75 a Purpuric rash.
    b Mononeuritis multiplex (possibly early sensorimotor polyneuropathy).
    c Polyarteritis nodosa.
    d i) Leucocytosis.
       ii) Raised ESR.
       iii) Positive hepatitis B surface antigen.

76 a i) Violaceous discolouration of skin of left cheek.
       ii) Depressed nasal bridge (a result of granulomatous destruction of the anterior nasal septum).
    b i) Sarcoidosis.
       ii) Tuberculosis.
    c Mantoux test.

77 a Delayed relaxation phase of the ankle jerk.
    b The serum thyroid stimulating hormone (TSH) level.

78 a Group A beta haemolytic streptococcal infection.
    b i) Acute rheumatic fever.
       ii) Acute glomerulonephritis (typically diffuse proliferative type).

79 a Inferior wall aneurysm.
    b Changes of full-thickness inferior/true posterior myocardial infarction:

Q waves in standard leads II, III, AVF, dominant R waves in the right-sided chest leads; persistent ST elevation in leads II, III and AVF; ST depression in the right sided chest leads.

  c The murmur of mitral incompetence may be heard if disruption to the posterior leaflet of the mitral valve has occurred.

80 a Koilonychia (spoon-shaped nails).
      b i)   Oesophageal web (Plummer-Vinson/Paterson-Kelly syndromes) in association with iron deficiency.
           ii)   Chronic blood loss from peptic or neoplastic oesophageal disease. (Oesophageal web itself predisposes to oesophageal carcinoma).

81 a Splenomegaly.
      b Splenomegaly makes 'idiopathic' thrombocytopenic purpura (ITP) very unlikely; and lymphoma, leukaemia, hypersplenism likely.
      c Normal. Megakaryocyte numbers may be increased. In ITP, thrombocytopenia follows peripheral autoimmune destruction of platelets.

82 a Herpes zoster ophthalmicus.
      b i)   Conjunctivitis, keratitis, iridocyclitis, optic neuritis (rarely).
           ii)   Encephalomyelitis.
           iii) Associated cranial nerve involvement (especially VIIth with facial palsy).
           iv) Secondary streptococcal/staphylococcal infection.
           v)   Haemorrhagic zoster (purpura fulminans).
           vi) Dissemination (immunosuppressed patients).
           vii) Post-herpetic neuralgia.

83 a Microaneurysms, dot and blot haemorrhages, hard exudates. Maculopathy.
      b Diabetes mellitus.

84 and 85
      a i) Striae.
          ii) Diffuse hyperpigmentation.
      b Right oculomotor (third cranial nerve) palsy.
      c Nelson's syndrome. (Pituitary corticotroph adenoma showing progressive growth after bilateral adrenalectomy for Cushing's disease. These tumours are often locally invasive).

86 a In most patients the abnormal cells are B lymphocytes but T-cell CLL may infrequently occur.
      b i)   Hypogammaglobulinaemia.
          ii) Monoclonal gammopathy.
      c i)   Bone marrow failure.
          ii) Autoimmune haemolytic anaemia.
      d None; there is no characteristic chromosomal abnormality.

87 a i) Heberden's nodes.
ii) Bouchard's nodes.
b Osteophytes.
(Occasionally joint effusions and painful cystic swelling adjacent to the joints may accompany rapidly developing Heberden's and Bouchard's nodes).

88 a Turner's syndrome.
b Features of aortic coarctation include,
i) Systemic hypertension.
ii) Inequality of radial pulses and of blood pressure in the arms (if the coarctation is proximal to the left subclavian artery — most are not).
iii) Radiofemoral delay.
iv) Scapular collateral vessels, with or without bruits.
v) Systolic murmur over the left upper chest (front and back).
vi) Systolic murmur from frequently associated bicuspid aortic valve.
vii) Left ventricular hypertrophy.

89 i) Fracture of the waist of the scaphoid.
ii) Bone density relatively greater in the scaphoid, suggesting avascular necrosis.

90 a i) Skin nodules.
ii) Café au lait patch.
iii) Axillary freckling (Crowe's sign).
b Neurofibromatosis (Von Recklinghausen's disease) — axillary freckling is said to be pathognomonic.

91 a Ringworm: spreading tinea cruris. Likely infecting organism tinea rubrum.
b Griseofulvin (orally).

92 a Skull base fracture involving the orbit with an expanding intracerebral (probably extradural) haematoma.
b Skull x-rays may demonstrate the fracture. Cerebral CT scan is the investigation of choice followed by neurosurgical intervention. "Blind" evacuation may be necessary if CT scanning is not available immediately.

93 a Prepatellar bursitis (housemaid's knee).
b None. It is a sterile inflammation due to trauma.

94 a Family history; predominantly proximal muscle weakness; absence of bulbar damage; absence of pyramidal signs.
b Physiotherapy. Swimming is particularly beneficial.

95 a A ganglion.
b Fibrous tissue of the joint capsule or tendon sheath.
c Traumatic obliteration (eg sharp blow) is associated with a high rate of recurrence. Excision is more likely to be successful.

96 and 97

    a Tuberous sclerosis (epiloia); adenoma sebaceum.

    b Leaf-shaped pale macules (a larger macule adjacent to the umbilicus, smaller lesions along the costal margins).

    c Nodules of glial proliferation usually on the surface of the cerebral cortex, gyri and ventricular surfaces.

    d i)   Shagreen patch.

        ii) Subungual fibroma

      (Café au lait spots, and pedunculated fibromata may also be found but are less typical).

98 a Left sided calcified pleural plaque.

    b Asbestos exposure (although pleural calcification can develop following any inflammatory pleural disease — e.g. empyema).

    c i)   Pulmonary fibrosis.

        ii) Bronchial carcinoma.

        iii) Pleural mesothelioma.

99 a Erythema ab igne.

    b Infra red radiation.

    c Yes. Epitheliomatous change has been described.

    d Hypothyroidism.

100 a Coloboma.

    b Congenital — defective closure of embryonic cleft.

    c May be associated with colobomata (of varying extent) of anterior uvea and adjacent retina.

101 a Pretibial myxoedema.

    b Graves' disease.

    c Corticosteroids i) under occlusive plastic dressing.

                      ii) injected intralesionally.

102 a Pityriasis versicolor.

    b Fungal infection — *pityrosoporum* species.

    c i)   Demonstration of ycasts and mycelia in scrapings.

        ii)   Pale yellow fluorescence under Wood's light.

103 a Herpes labialis (cold sores).

    b Herpes simplex virus type 1.

    c Commonly associated with underlying bacterial infection

      eg. lobar pneumonia

         bacterial meningitis.

104 a Autosomal dominant.

    b Epilepsy.

105 and 106

    a Violaceous flat-topped polygonal papules.

    b Lichen planus.

    c Epitheliomatous transformation may occur in ulcerative mouth lesions.

107 Blindness in his left eye due to ischaemic optic atrophy. Cholesterol crystals and mural plaques can be seen in the upper nasal quadrant.

108 a Herpes zoster ophthalmicus.
      b It indicates that the cornea and uveal tract may be involved.
      c Acyclovir, vidarabine, or idoxuridine will limit viral replication. Systemic corticosteroids may reduce the incidence of post herpetic neuralgia but are contraindicated in the immunocompromised host. Local corticosteroids and atropine may be useful if anteror uveitis has developed.

109 a i)   Extensive soft tissue calcification.
          ii)   Cardiomegaly.
      b Dermatomyositis.

110 a Urticaria pigmentosa.
      b Abnormal proliferation of mast cells.
      c Mast cell degranulation, with release of vasoactive peptides (histamine, kinins).
      d Codeine phosphate, alcohol (also salicyclic acid, polymixin B).

111 a Keratoacanthoma.
      b Squamous carcinoma.

112 and 113
      a i)   Perianal disease — fistulae, fissures, skin tags.
         ii) Erythema nodosum.
      b Crohn's disease.
      c i)   Ulcerative colitis.
         ii) Yersinia, salmonella, campylobacter enteritides.
         iii) Tuberculosis.
         iv) Sarcoidosis (liver, salivary glands may be affected).

114 a Pruritus.
      b Cholestyramine.

115 a Pigment disturbance and exudation adjacent to and encroaching on the macula.
      b Senile macular degeneration.
      c Choroid.

116 a Swelling behind left sternomastoid.
      b Left Horner's syndrome secondary to cervical mass.
      c She has developed gastric carcinoma as a complication of long-standing pernicious anaemia, with resultant cervical lymphadenopathy (Troisier's sign).

117 a Ehlers Danlos syndrome
    b i)   Skin hyperelasticity.
       ii)   Skin and blood vessel fragility. (Easy bruising and delayed skin healing with papyraceous scars and molluscoid pseudotumours.)
       iii) Joint hyperextensibility — flat feet, genu recurvatum, kyphoscoliosis.
       iv) Characteristic facies — wide nasal bridge, hypertelorism, epicanthic folds.
       v)   Occasionally, retinal angioid streaks, blue sclerae, aortic dissection.

118 a Beau's line.
    b When isolated to one nail, local injury is the likely cause. When all nails are affected, these indicate recent systemic illness interfering with nail growth temporarily (eg. measles, mumps, pneumonia, coronary thrombosis).

119 a Sabre tibiae.
    b i)   Paget's disease.
       ii)   Congenital syphilis.
    c Osteogenic sarcoma, complicating Paget's disease.

120 and 121
    a Arachnodactyly.
    b Subluxation of the lens (upwards).
    c Marfan's syndrome: autosomal dominant.
    d Homocystinuria (in this condition the lens is said typically to sublux downwards).

122 a Palmar erythema.
    b i)   Cirrhosis (especially alcoholic).
       ii)   Normal pregnancy.
       iii) Rheumatoid arthritis.
       iv) Thyrotoxicosis.
       v)   Dermatological disorders — eczema, psoriasis, pityriasis rubra pilaris
          Others include polycythaemia, diabetes mellitus, mitral valve disease, beri-beri. May occasionally be inherited.

123 Post-herpetic neuralgia.

124 and 125
    a Calcaneal spurs.
    b Reiter's disease.

126 a Band keratopathy.
    b Parathyroid exploration/parathyroidectomy.

127 a i)   Infected branchial cyst.
       ii)   Tuberculous lymphadenopathy/abscess.
    b i)   Clinical: infected branchial cyst tends to cause sternomastoid

spasm. Tuberculosis tends to cause fixation to the overlying tissues.

ii) Aspiration, microscopy, culture (+ additional evidence of tuberculosis: Mantoux, chest x-ray).

128 a 'Senile' cataract.
   b Diabetes mellitus.
   c These include:
   i) Refractory disturbances — hypermetropia with rising blood glucose; myopia with falling blood glucose.
   ii) Rubeosis iridis.
   iii) Retinopathy — background, proliferative.
   iv) Intrinsic and extrinsic ocular muscle paralysis (cranial nerve lesions and autonomic neuropathy).

129 a i) Type II diabetes mellitus.
   ii) Mental retardation.
   iii) Hypogonadism.
   iv) Muscle hypotonia.
   b i) Laurence-Moon-Biedl syndrome (polydactyly, retinitis pigmentosa).
   ii) Alstrom syndrome (nerve deafness).
   iii) Biemond syndrome (polydactyly, iris colobomata).

130 a Complete heart block with a high nodal escape rhythm. The QRS complex is normal.
   b Congenital.
   c His bundle electrocardiography.
   d None.

131 a Papilloedema with peripapillary flame haemorrhages.
   b Acute mountain sickness leading to cerebral oedema.
   c Immediate descent. Delay may be fatal.

132 a Thyroglossal cyst.
   b None; it arises from a downgrowth of endoderm in the midline.

133 a Oval macrocytes; hypersegmented polymorphonuclear leukocytes.
   b Subacute degeneration of the spinal cord due to vitamin B12 deficiency.
   c Optic atrophy; spastic paraplegia; mental changes including depression, dementia, confusional psychosis; peripheral neuropathy.

134 a i) Right ptosis.
   ii) Right miosis.
   iii) Sutured laceration overlying sternomastoid and the right anterior triangle.
   b Horner's syndrome due to damage to the cervical sympathetic fibres.

135 a i) Intrinsic muscle wasting (most noticeably of first dorsal interossei).

ii) Prominent ulnar styloids.
iii) Prominent metacarpal heads.
iv) Ulnar deviation at the metacarpophalangeal joints (especially of left hand).
v) 'Z' deformity of left thumb.
b Rheumatoid arthritis.
c Rupture of the extensor digitorum tendons (third, fourth, fifth).

136 a There are bilateral nodular opacities, most marked in the lower and mid zones.
b i) Pulmonary function tests may show a restrictive ventilatory defect with reduced transfer factor, hypoxaemia and hypocapnia.
ii) Precipitating antibodies to avian protein may be detected.
iii) Provocation testing may reproduce the symptoms and support the diagnosis.
c Examples include: farmer's lung; bagassosis (sugar cane); byssinosis (cotton); cheese washer's lung; coffee worker's lung; detergent worker's lung; maltworker's lung; maple-bark worker's lung; mushroom worker's lung; prawnworker's lung; suberosis (cork); woodworker's lung.

137 This includes
i) Femoral hernia.
ii) Ectopic testis.
iii) Femoral lymphadenopathy.
iv) Saphena varix.
v) Psoas abscess.
vi) Femoral aneurysm.

138 1 Carina with right and left main bronchi.
2 Descending thoracic aorta.
3 Bulla in left lung.
4 Normal left lung parenchyma.
5 Normal right lung with small emphysematous bullae throughout the parenchyma.

139, 140, 141 and 142
a Psoriasis.
b i) Elephantine ('psoriasis inveterata').
ii) Flexural/intertriginous.
iii) Pustular.
iv) Nummular (the commonest form).

143 a Xanthomata.
b Primary biliary cirrhosis.
c Antimitochondrial antibody (A.M.A.). Presence of A.M.A. makes extrahepatic biliary obstruction unlikely.

144 a Ophthalmic Graves' disease.
Upward gaze is most typically impaired in this condition, owing to oedema and to lymphocytic and fatty infiltration of the orbital

contents, particularly of the extra ocular muscles.

b Radioactive iodine.

c Infiltrative eye disease may occur irrespective of thyroid status. Post-radioactive iodine hypothyroidism, however, is most likely to induce progressive eye changes.

145 a Scrofula — tuberculous cervical lymphadenitis.

    b i)   Biopsy — histological evidence of tuberculosis.

      ii)   Bacteriological culture — but isolation rate of mycobacterium tuberculosis is only about 60%.

    c Anti-tuberculosis chemotherapy.

      eg. Rifampicin.

          Ethambutol.

          Isoniazid.

146 a i)   Wasting of left sternomastoid.

      ii)   Loss of action of left trapezius.

    b Left XIth cranial (accessory) nerve paralysis.

147 and 148

    a Bronchiectasis with hypertrophic pulmonary osteoarthropathy.

    b Periosteal elevation with new bone formation.

    c Primary intrathoracic malignancy is the commonest association. Other causes include lung abscess, empyema, cyanotic congenital heart disease, cirrhosis and inflammatory bowel disease.

149 a Jaundice.

    b Hypoglycaemia or alcohol withdrawal if the patient was alcoholic.

    c Fresh frozen plasma will be more effective than vitamin K.

    d The ocular signs suggest Wernicke's encephalopathy rather than delirium tremens or hepatic encephalopathy, and may have been precipitated by the glucose infusion. Thiamine should have been given beforehand.

150 a Widening of the sutures; multiple sutural (Wormian) bones.

    b Hypothyroidism.

    c No.

151 a Hypothyroidism.

    b She is hypercarotenaemic (incidentally she was found to have an associated vitamin B_{12} deficiency).

152 a He has developed cryoglobulinaemia.

    b Raynaud's phenomenon; livedo reticularis; digital ulceration.

    c Protection of the extremities from cold; specific treatment of the underlying myeloma; plasmapheresis is of particular benefit if the cryoglobulin is IgM.

    d Blood should be taken and maintained at 37° to allow the detection of cryoglobulins.

153 and 154
    a i) Knuckle pigmentation.
      ii) Adrenal calcification.
    b Primary adrenal insufficiency; tuberculosis.

155 a Ascites.
    b Paracentesis.
    c i) Alcohol.
      ii) Drugs — e.g. diuretics, narcotics.
      iii) Gastrointestinal haemorrhage.
      iv) Infection.
      v) Surgery (especially portacaval shunting).

156 a Priapism.
    b i) Chronic granulocytic leukaemia.
      ii) Spinal cord injury.
      iii) Sickle-cell anaemia.

157 and 158
    a Pyoderma gangrenosum
    b Ulcerative colitis.

159 a Nephrotic syndrome. Her serum calcium, corrected for hypoalbuminaemia, is normal.
    b 'Minimal change' nephropathy, on renal biopsy.

160 a Osler's nodes (tender; appear typically in finger and toe pulps, thenar and hypothenar eminences).
    b Infective endocarditis.
    c i) Janeway lesions (non-tender; appear typically on the palms and soles).
      ii) Splinter haemorrhages.
      iii) Conjunctival haemorrhages.
      iv) Roth's spots (fundal haemorrhages with central pallor).
      v) Changing cardiac murmurs.
      vi) Finger clubbing.
      vii) Splenomegaly.
      viii) Pallor.
    The typical triad of infective endocarditis includes fever, 'embolic' phenomena and changing murmurs.

161 i) Reticulohistiocytosis.
    ii) Gout.

162 a Target lesions.
    b Erythema multiforme.
    c i) Herpes simplex.
      ii) Mycoplasma pneumonia.

163 a Right oculomotor (third cranial nerve) palsy.
    b The pupillary fibres lying peripherally in the nerve are supplied by pial

blood vessels and so tend to be spared in ischaemic oculomotor palsies.

164 a Rheumatoid arthritis.
   b A shoe insole should be fitted. This should be modelled to provide support behind the metatarsal heads, thus taking weight off them.

165 and 166
   a i)   Bilateral hilar lymphadenopathy.
     ii) Nodular infiltrates in both lung fields, predominantly in the lower zones.
   b Numerous punched out lytic defects; lacework reticulated pattern in the phalanges; some resorption of the distal phalanges.
   c Sarcoidosis.

167 and 168
   a Measles.
   b i)   Koplik's spots.
     ii) They develop in the prodrome.
   c Lymphoid hyperplasia with multinucleate giant cells (Warthin-Finkeldey cells).

169 a A — Common bile duct.
      B — Gall stone.
      C — Portal vein.
      D — Inferior vena cava.
   b i)   Endoscopic retrograde cholangiopancreatography.
     ii) Percutaneous transhepatic cholangiogram.
     iii) Intravenous cholangiogram. This is unlikely to demonstrate the biliary system unless jaundice is mild and/or resolving.

170 and 171
   a Vasculitis (causing ulceration, purpura).
   b These include
     i)   Rheumatoid nodules.
     ii) Digital arteritic infarcts (usually around and under the nails, finger pulps: occasionally bullous, may become gangrenous).
     iii) Livedo reticularis.
        Neuropathic ulceration may occur secondary to vasculitic sensory neuropathy. Gravitational ulcers are more common in rheumatoid disease. Pyoderma gangrenosum has been described.

172 a Absent axillary hair.
   b Sheehan's syndrome (post-partum pituitary necrosis).
   c i)   Failure of postpartum breast engorgement and lactation.
     ii) Failure of (shaved) pubic hair to regrow, failed growth/loss of axillary hair.
     iii) Continued amenorrhoea.
        (Other features of pituitary failure, eg hypothyroidism, if present at all, are usually late in onset).

173 a Scarring alopecia.
     b i)   Secondary or tertiary syphilis (although the degree of alopecia
              seen here is rather extensive for secondary syphilis).
        ii) Systemic lupus erythematosus.
        iii) Leprosy.
    In ii) and iii), the VDRL test is falsely positive.

174 and 175
     a Granuloma annulare.
     b Diabetes mellitus.

176 a Atrial flutter with 2:1 block.
     b Beat to beat variation in intensity of the first heart sound occurs in
        atrial flutter.
     c Increase in the degree of AV block; and conversion to atrial
        fibrillation commonly occurs.

177 and 178
     a Perforating foot ulcer; gas in the soft tissues of the foot.
     b Diabetes mellitus resulting in a neuropathic ulcer with superinfection
        by gas-producing organisms.
     c Clostridium species or E. coli are the major causes of this appearance.

179 Degenerative disease of the lumbar spine. Ankylosing spondylitis may
    give rise to identical symptoms and signs, but is unlikely to present at
    this age.

180 a Loss of central vision with preservation of peripheral vision.
     b Congenital toxoplasmosis. Syphilis, toxocariasis or rubella are
        unlikely to cause such a well-defined, pigmented lesion.
     c No. Subsequent pregnancies are not affected.

181 and 182
     a Acute myeloblastic leukaemia, promyelocytic variant.
     b Disseminated intravascular coagulation.

183 a Subarachnoid haemorrhage with blood extending into the third and
        lateral ventricles.
     b Rupture of an aneurysm of the anterior communicating artery.

184 a The tympanic membrane is opaque and retracted, with a horizontal
        fluid level. Chronic secretory otitis media.
     b Bilaterally negative Rinne tests; Weber's test may lateralise if the
        severity of disease is unequal.
     c No. Autoinflation, Politzerisation, decongestants and myringotomy
        with or without grommet insertion are the basis of treatment.

185 a Bilateral ptosis, more marked on the left.
     b Myasthenia gravis.
     c Intravenous injection of edrophonium chloride.
     d No. Peak incidence in men is in the sixth and seventh decades.

186 a Pigmentation of the lips.
 b Gastrointestinal polyposis; Peutz-Jegher syndrome.
 c The risk of malignant change in the polyps is very low but such change has been recorded. In women, there is an increased incidence of ovarian carcinoma.

187 a Massive hilar, paratracheal and upper mediastinal lymphadenopathy.
 b Hodgkin's disease.
 c Nodular sclerosing (the most frequent variety overall).

188 a Knuckle (Garrod's) pads on the middle and ring fingers.
 b It may be inherited as an autosomal dominant condition or may arise spontaneously.
 c Dupuytren's contractures.

189 and 190
 a i) 'Calabar' swelling of left hand.
   ii) Soft tissue calcification.
 b Loiasis — caused by the filarial parasite loa loa.
 c Confined to Central Africa.

191 a Urticaria (with annular lesions).
 b i) Blood transfusion.
   ii) Dextran (40 or 70) transfusion.

192 a Iridodialysis.
 b i) Penetrating eye injury.
   ii) Surgery (eg. for glaucoma).

193 a Central cyanosis due to methaemoglobinaemia.
 b Sodium or potassium chlorate.
 c Intravenous methylene blue.

194 a Mumps meningitis.
 b Clear cerebrospinal fluid under normal pressure with a lymphocytosis, normal glucose and moderately elevated protein.
 c Paired serology to mumps S and V antigens.

INDEX

TABLETS

PLENDIL®

(FELODIPINE, MSD)

EXTENDED-RELEASE TABLETS

DESCRIPTION

PLENDIL* (Felodipine, MSD) is a calcium antagonist (calcium channel blocker). Felodipine is a dihydropyridine derivative that is chemically described as ± ethyl methyl 4-(2,3-dichlorophenyl)-1, 4-dihydro-2,6-dimethyl-3,5-pyridinedicarboxylate. Its empirical formula is $C_{18}H_{19}Cl_2NO_4$ and its structural formula is:

Felodipine is a slightly yellowish, crystalline powder with a molecular weight of 384.26. It is insoluble in water and is freely soluble in dichloromethane and ethanol. Felodipine is a racemic mixture.

Tablets PLENDIL provide extended release of felodipine. They are available as tablets containing 5 mg or 10 mg of felodipine for oral administration. In addition to the active ingredient felodipine, each tablet contains the following inactive ingredients: cellulose, iron oxides, lactose, polyethylene glycol, sodium stearyl fumarate, titanium dioxide and other ingredients.

CLINICAL PHARMACOLOGY

Mechanism of Action

Felodipine is a member of the dihydropyridine class of calcium channel antagonists (calcium channel blockers). It reversibly competes with nitrendipine and/or other calcium channel blockers for dihydropyridine binding sites, blocks voltage-dependent Ca + + currents in vascular smooth muscle and cultured rabbit atrial cells and blocks potassium-induced contracture of the rat portal vein.

In vitro studies show that the effects of felodipine on contractile processes are selective, with greater effects on vascular smooth muscle than cardiac muscle. Negative inotropic effects can be detected *in vitro*, but such effects have not been seen in intact animals.

The effect of felodipine on blood pressure is principally a consequence of a dose-related decrease of peripheral vascular resistance in man, with a modest reflex increase in heart rate (see *Cardiovascular Effects*). With the exception of a mild diuretic effect seen in several animal species and man, the effects of felodipine are accounted for by its effects on peripheral vascular resistance.

Pharmacokinetics and Metabolism

Following oral administration, felodipine is almost completely absorbed and undergoes extensive first-pass metabolism. The systemic bioavailability of PLENDIL is approximately 20 percent. Mean peak concentrations following the administration of PLENDIL are reached in 2.5 to 5 hours. Both peak plasma concentration and the area under the plasma concentration time curve (AUC) increase linearly with doses up to 20 mg. Felodipine is greater than 99 percent bound to plasma proteins.

Following intravenous administration, the plasma concentration of felodipine declined triexponentially with mean disposition half-lives of 4.8 minutes, 1.5 hours and 9.1 hours. The mean contributions of the three individual

PLENDIL®
(Felodipine, MSD)
Extended-Release Tablets

phases to the overall AUC were 15, 40 and 45 percent, respectively, in the order of increasing $t_\frac{1}{2}$.

Following oral administration of the immediate-release formulation, the plasma level of felodipine also declined polyexponentially with a mean terminal $t_\frac{1}{2}$ of 11 to 16 hours. The mean peak and trough steady-state plasma concentrations achieved after 10 mg of the immediate-release formulation given once a day to normal volunteers, were 20 and 0.5 nmol/L, respectively. The trough plasma concentration of felodipine in most individuals was substantially below the concentration needed to effect a half-maximal decline in blood pressure (EC_{50}) [4-6 nmol/L for felodipine], thus precluding once a day dosing with the immediate-release formulation.

Following administration of a 10-mg dose of PLENDIL, the extended-release formulation, to young, healthy volunteers, mean peak and trough steady-state plasma concentrations of felodipine were 7 and 2 nmol/L, respectively. Corresponding values in hypertensive patients (mean age 64) after a 20-mg dose of PLENDIL were 23 and 7 nmol/L. Since the EC_{50} for felodipine is 4 to 6 nmol/L, a 5 to 10-mg dose of PLENDIL in some patients, and a 20-mg dose in others, would be expected to provide an antihypertensive effect that persists for 24 hours (see *Cardiovascular Effects* below and DOSAGE AND ADMINISTRATION).

The systemic plasma clearance of felodipine in young healthy subjects is about 0.8 L/min and the apparent volume of distribution is about 10 L/kg.

Following an oral or intravenous dose of ^{14}C-labeled felodipine in man, about 70 percent of the dose of radioactivity was recovered in urine and 10 percent in the feces. A negligible amount of intact felodipine is recovered in the urine and feces (<0.5%). Six metabolites, which account for 23 percent of the oral dose, have been identified; none has significant vasodilating activity.

Following administration of PLENDIL to hypertensive patients, mean peak plasma concentrations at steady state are about 20 percent higher than after a single dose. Blood pressure response is correlated with plasma concentrations of felodipine.

The bioavailability of PLENDIL is not influenced by the presence of food in the gastrointestinal tract. In a study of six patients, the bioavailability of felodipine was increased more than two-fold when taken with doubly concentrated grapefruit juice, compared to when taken with water or orange juice. A similar finding has been seen with some other dihydropyridine calcium antagonists, but to a lesser extent than that seen with felodipine.

Age Effects: Plasma concentrations of felodipine, after a single dose and at steady state, increase with age. Mean clearance of felodipine in elderly hypertensives (mean age 74) was only 45 percent of that of young volunteers (mean age 26). At steady state mean AUC for young patients was 39 percent of that for the elderly. Data for intermediate age ranges suggest that the AUCs fall between the extremes of the young and the elderly.

Hepatic Dysfunction: In patients with hepatic disease, the clearance of felodipine was reduced to about 60 percent of that seen in normal young volunteers.

Renal impairment does not alter the plasma concentration profile of felodipine; although higher concentrations of the metabolites are present in the plasma due to decreased urinary excretion, these are inactive.

1

PLENDIL®
(Felodipine, MSD)
Extended-Release Tablets

Animal studies have demonstrated that felodipine crosses the blood-brain barrier and the placenta.

Cardiovascular Effects

Following administration of PLENDIL, a reduction in blood pressure generally occurs within two to five hours. During chronic administration, substantial blood pressure control lasts for 24 hours, with trough reductions in diastolic blood pressure approximately 40-50 percent of peak reductions. The antihypertensive effect is dose-dependent and correlates with the plasma concentration of felodipine.

A reflex increase in heart rate frequently occurs during the first week of therapy; this increase attenuates over time. Heart rate increases of 5-10 beats per minute may be seen during chronic dosing. The increase is inhibited by beta-blocking agents.

The P-R interval of the ECG is not affected by felodipine when administered alone or in combination with a beta-blocking agent. Felodipine alone or in combination with a beta-blocking agent has been shown, in clinical and electrophysiologic studies, to have no significant effect on cardiac conduction (P-R, P-Q and H-V intervals).

In clinical trials in hypertensive patients without clinical evidence of left ventricular dysfunction, no symptoms suggestive of a negative inotropic effect were noted; however none would be expected in this population (see PRECAUTIONS).

Renal/Endocrine Effects

Renal vascular resistance is decreased by felodipine while glomerular filtration rate remains unchanged. Mild diuresis, natriuresis and kaliuresis have been observed during the first week of therapy. No significant effects on serum electrolytes were observed during short- and long-term therapy.

In clinical trials increases in plasma noradrenaline levels have been observed.

Clinical Studies

Felodipine produces dose-related decreases in systolic and diastolic blood pressure as demonstrated in six placebo-controlled, dose response studies using either immediate-release or extended-release dosage forms. These studies enrolled over 800 patients on active treatment, at total daily doses ranging from 2.5 to 20 mg. In those studies felodipine was administered either as monotherapy or was added to beta blockers. The results of the two studies with PLENDIL given once daily as monotherapy are shown in the table below:

MEAN REDUCTIONS IN BLOOD PRESSURE (mmHg)*
Systolic/Diastolic

Dose	N	Mean Peak Response	Mean Trough Response	Trough/Peak Ratios (%s)
Study 1 (8 weeks)				
2.5 mg	68	9.4/4.7	2.7/2.5	29/53
5 mg	69	9.5/6.3	2.4/3.7	25/59
10 mg	67	18.0/10.8	10.0/6.0	56/56
Study 2 (4 weeks)				
10 mg	50	5.3/7.2	1.5/3.2	33/40**
20 mg	50	11.3/10.2	4.5/3.2	43/34**

*Placebo response subtracted
**Different number of patients available for peak and trough measurements

INDICATIONS AND USAGE

PLENDIL is indicated for the treatment of hypertension. PLENDIL may be used alone or concomitantly with other antihypertensive agents.

CONTRAINDICATIONS

PLENDIL is contraindicated in patients who are hypersensitive to this product.

PRECAUTIONS

General

Hypotension: Felodipine, like other calcium antagonists, may occasionally precipitate significant hypotension and rarely syncope. It may lead to reflex tachycardia which in susceptible individuals may precipitate angina pectoris. (See ADVERSE REACTIONS.)

Heart Failure: Although acute hemodynamic studies in a small number of patients with NYHA Class II or III heart failure treated with felodipine have not demonstrated negative inotropic effects, safety in patients with heart failure has not been established. Caution therefore should be exercised when using PLENDIL in patients with heart failure or compromised ventricular function, particularly in combination with a beta blocker.

Elderly Patients or Patients with Impaired Liver Function: Patients over 65 years of age or patients with impaired liver function may have elevated plasma concentrations of felodipine and may therefore respond to lower doses of PLENDIL. These patients should have their blood pressure monitored closely during dosage adjustment of PLENDIL and should rarely require doses above 10 mg. (See CLINICAL PHARMACOLOGY and DOSAGE AND ADMINISTRATION.)

Peripheral Edema: Peripheral edema, generally mild and not associated with generalized fluid retention, was the most common adverse event in the clinical trials. The incidence of peripheral edema was both dose- and age-dependent. Frequency of peripheral edema ranged from about 10 percent in patients under 50 years of age taking 5 mg daily to about 30 percent in those over 60 years of age taking 20 mg daily. This adverse effect generally occurs within 2-3 weeks of the initiation of treatment.

Information for Patients

Patients should be instructed to take PLENDIL whole and not to crush or chew the tablets. They should be told that mild gingival hyperplasia (gum swelling) has been reported. Good dental hygiene decreases its incidence and severity.

NOTE: As with many other drugs, certain advice to patients being treated with PLENDIL is warranted. This information is intended to aid in the safe and effective use of this medication. It is not a disclosure of all possible adverse or intended effects.

Drug Interactions

Beta-Blocking Agents: A pharmacokinetic study of felodipine in conjunction with metoprolol demonstrated no significant effects on the pharmacokinetics of felodipine. The AUC and C_{max} of metoprolol, however, were increased approximately 31 and 38 percent, respectively. In controlled clinical trials, however, beta blockers including metoprolol were concurrently administered with felodipine and were well tolerated.

Cimetidine: In healthy subjects pharmacokinetic studies showed an approximately 50 percent increase in the area under the plasma concentration time curve (AUC) as well as the C_{max} of felodipine when given concomitantly with cimetidine. It is anticipated that a clinically significant interaction may occur in some hypertensive patients. Therefore, it is recommended that low doses of PLENDIL be used when given concomitantly with cimetidine.

Digoxin: When given concomitantly with felodipine the peak plasma concentration of digoxin was significantly increased. There was, however, no significant change in the AUC of digoxin.

Other Concomitant Therapy: In healthy subjects there were no clinically significant interac-

2

tions when felodipine was given concomitantly with indomethacin or spironolactone.

Interaction with Food: See CLINICAL PHARMACOLOGY, *Pharmacokinetics and Metabolism.*

Carcinogenesis, Mutagenesis, Impairment of Fertility
In a two-year carcinogenicity study in rats fed felodipine at doses of 7.7, 23.1 or 69.3 mg/kg/day (up to 28 times* the maximum recommended human dose on a mg/m² basis), a dose-related increase in the incidence of benign interstitial cell tumors of the testes (Leydig cell tumors) was observed in treated male rats. These tumors were not observed in a similar study in mice at doses up to 138.6 mg/kg/day (28 times* the maximum recommended human dose on a mg/m² basis). Felodipine, at the doses employed in the two-year rat study, has been shown to lower testicular testosterone and to produce a corresponding increase in serum luteinizing hormone in rats. The Leydig cell tumor development is possibly secondary to these hormonal effects which have not been observed in man.

In this same rat study a dose-related increase in the incidence of focal squamous cell hyperplasia compared to control was observed in the esophageal groove of male and female rats in all dose groups. No other drug-related esophageal or gastric pathology was observed in the rats or with chronic administration in mice and dogs. The latter species, like man, has no anatomical structure comparable to the esophageal groove.

Felodipine was not carcinogenic when fed to mice at doses of up to 138.6 mg/kg/day (28 times* the maximum recommended human dose on a mg/m² basis) for periods of up to 80 weeks in males and 99 weeks in females.

Felodipine did not display any mutagenic activity *in vitro* in the Ames microbial mutagenicity test or in the mouse lymphoma forward mutation assay. No clastogenic potential was seen *in vivo* in the mouse micronucleus test at oral doses up to 2500 mg/kg (506 times* the maximum recommended human dose on a mg/m² basis) or *in vitro* in a human lymphocyte chromosome aberration assay.

A fertility study in which male and female rats were administered doses of 3.8, 9.6 or 26.9 mg/kg/day showed no significant effect of felodipine on reproductive performance.

Pregnancy
Pregnancy Category C
Teratogenic Effects: Studies in pregnant rabbits administered doses of 0.46, 1.2, 2.3 and 4.6 mg/kg/day (from 0.4 to 4 times* the maximum recommended human dose on a mg/m² basis) showed digital anomalies consisting of reduction in size and degree of ossification of the terminal phalanges in the fetuses. The frequency and severity of the changes appeared dose-related and were noted even at the lowest dose. These changes have been shown to occur with other members of the dihydropyridine class and are possibly a result of compromised uterine blood flow. Similar fetal anomalies were not observed in rats given felodipine.

In a teratology study in cynomolgus monkeys no reduction in the size of the terminal phalanges was observed but an abnormal position of the distal phalanges was noted in about 40 percent of the fetuses.

Nonteratogenic Effects: A prolongation of parturition with difficult labor and an increased frequency of fetal and early postnatal deaths were observed in rats administered doses of 9.6

mg/kg/day (4 times* the maximum human dose on a mg/m² basis) and above.

Significant enlargement of the mammary glands in excess of the normal enlargement for pregnant rabbits was found with doses greater than or equal to 1.2 mg/kg/day (equal to the maximum human dose on a mg/m² basis). This effect occurred only in pregnant rabbits and regressed during lactation. Similar changes in the mammary glands were not observed in rats or monkeys.

There are no adequate and well-controlled studies in pregnant women. If felodipine is used during pregnancy, or if the patient becomes pregnant while taking this drug, she should be apprised of the potential hazard to the fetus, possible digital anomalies of the infant, and the potential effects of felodipine on labor and delivery, and on the mammary glands of pregnant females.

Nursing Mothers
It is not known whether this drug is secreted in human milk and because of the potential for serious adverse reactions from felodipine in the infant, a decision should be made whether to discontinue nursing or to discontinue the drug, taking into account the importance of the drug to the mother.

Pediatric Use
Safety and effectiveness in children have not been established.

ADVERSE REACTIONS

In controlled studies in the United States and overseas approximately 3000 patients were treated with felodipine as either the extended-release or the immediate-release formulation.

The most common clinical adverse experiences reported with PLENDIL administered as monotherapy in all settings and with all dosage forms of felodipine were peripheral edema and headache. Peripheral edema was generally mild, but it was age- and dose-related and resulted in discontinuation of therapy in about 4 percent of the enrolled patients. Discontinuation of therapy due to any clinical adverse experience occurred in about 9 percent of the patients receiving PLENDIL, principally for peripheral edema, headache, or flushing.

Adverse experiences that occurred with an incidence of 1.5 percent or greater during monotherapy with PLENDIL without regard to causality are compared to placebo in the table below.

Percent of Patients with Adverse Effects in Controlled
Trials of PLENDIL as Monotherapy
(Incidence of discontinuations shown in parentheses)

Adverse Effect	PLENDIL % N = 730		Placebo % N = 283
Peripheral Edema	22.3	(4.2)	3.5
Headache	18.6	(2.1)	10.6
Flushing	6.4	(1.0)	1.1
Dizziness	5.8	(0.8)	3.2
Upper Respiratory Infection	5.5	(0.1)	1.1
Asthenia	4.7	(0.1)	2.8
Cough	2.9	(0.0)	0.4
Paresthesia	2.5	(0.1)	1.8
Dyspepsia	2.3	(0.0)	1.4
Chest Pain	2.1	(0.1)	1.4
Nausea	1.9	(0.8)	1.1
Muscle Cramps	1.9	(0.0)	1.1
Palpitation	1.8	(0.5)	2.5
Abdominal Pain	1.8	(0.3)	1.1
Constipation	1.6	(0.1)	1.1
Diarrhea	1.6	(0.1)	1.1
Pharyngitis	1.6	(0.0)	0.4
Rhinorrhea	1.6	(0.0)	0.0
Back Pain	1.6	(0.0)	1.1
Rash	1.5	(0.1)	1.1

---

*Based on patient weight of 50 kg

In the two dose response studies using PLENDIL as monotherapy, the following table describes the incidence (percent) of adverse experiences that were dose-related:

Adverse Effect	Placebo N = 121	2.5 mg N = 71	5.0 mg N = 72	10.0 mg N = 123	20 mg N = 50
Peripheral Edema	2.5	1.4	13.9	19.5	36.0
Palpitation	0.8	1.4	0.0	2.4	12.0
Headache	12.4	11.3	11.1	18.7	28.0
Flushing	0.0	4.2	2.8	8.1	20.0

In addition, adverse experiences that occurred in 0.5 up to 1.5 percent of patients who received PLENDIL in all controlled clinical studies (listed in order of decreasing severity within each category) and serious adverse events that occurred at a lower rate or were found during marketing experience (those lower rate events are in italics) were: *Body as a Whole:* Facial edema, warm sensation; *Cardiovascular:* Tachycardia, *myocardial infarction, hypotension, syncope, angina pectoris,* arrhythmia; *Digestive:* Vomiting, dry mouth, flatulence; *Hematologic: Anemia; Musculoskeletal:* Arthralgia, arm pain, knee pain, leg pain, foot pain, hip pain, myalgia; *Nervous/Psychiatric:* Depression, anxiety disorders, insomnia, irritability, nervousness, somnolence; *Respiratory:* Bronchitis, influenza, sinusitis, dyspnea, epistaxis, respiratory infection, sneezing; *Skin:* Contusion, erythema, urticaria; *Urogenital:* Decreased libido, impotence, urinary frequency, urinary urgency, dysuria.

Felodipine, as an immediate release formulation, has also been studied as monotherapy in 680 patients with hypertension in U.S. and overseas controlled clinical studies. Other adverse experiences not listed above and with an incidence of 0.5 percent or greater include: *Body as a Whole:* Fatigue; *Digestive:* Gastrointestinal pain; *Musculoskeletal:* Arthritis, local weakness, neck pain, shoulder pain, ankle pain; *Nervous/Psychiatric:* Tremor; *Respiratory:* Rhinitis; *Skin:* Hyperhidrosis, pruritus; *Special Senses:* Blurred vision, tinnitus; *Urogenital:* Nocturia.

Gingival Hyperplasia: Gingival hyperplasia, usually mild, occurred in <0.5 percent of patients in controlled studies. This condition may be avoided or may regress with improved dental hygiene. (See PRECAUTIONS, *Information for Patients.*)

Clinical Laboratory Test Findings

Serum Electrolytes: No significant effects on serum electrolytes were observed during short- and long-term therapy (see CLINICAL PHARMACOLOGY, *Renal/Endocrine Effects*).

Serum Glucose: No significant effects on fasting serum glucose were observed in patients treated with PLENDIL in the U.S. controlled study.

Liver Enzymes: One of two episodes of elevated serum transaminases decreased once drug was discontinued in clinical studies; no follow-up was available for the other patient.

OVERDOSAGE

Oral doses of 240 mg/kg and 264 mg/kg in male and female mice, respectively and 2390 mg/kg and 2250 mg/kg in male and female rats, respectively, caused significant lethality.

In a suicide attempt, one patient took 150 mg felodipine together with 15 tablets each of atenolol and spironolactone and 20 tablets of nitrazepam. The patient's blood pressure and heart rate were normal on admission to hospital; he subsequently recovered without significant sequelae.

Overdosage might be expected to cause excessive peripheral vasodilation with marked hypotension and possibly bradycardia.

If severe hypotension occurs, symptomatic treatment should be instituted. The patient should be placed supine with the legs elevated. The administration of intravenous fluids may be useful to treat hypotension due to overdosage with calcium antagonists. In case of accompanying bradycardia, atropine (0.5-1 mg) should be administered intravenously. Sympathomimetic drugs may also be given if the physician feels they are warranted.

It has not been established whether felodipine can be removed from the circulation by hemodialysis.

DOSAGE AND ADMINISTRATION

The recommended initial dose is 5 mg once a day. Therapy should be adjusted individually according to patient response, generally at intervals of not less than two weeks. The usual dosage range is 5-10 mg once daily. The maximum recommended daily dose is 20 mg once a day. That dose in clinical trials showed an increased blood pressure response but a large increase in the rate of peripheral edema and other vasodilatory adverse events (see ADVERSE REACTIONS). Modification of the recommended dosage is usually not required in patients with renal impairment.

PLENDIL should be swallowed whole and not crushed or chewed.

Use in the Elderly or Patients with Impaired Liver Function: Patients over 65 years of age or patients with impaired liver function, because they may develop higher plasma concentrations of felodipine, should have their blood pressure monitored closely during dosage adjustment (see PRECAUTIONS). In general, doses above 10 mg should not be considered in these patients.

HOW SUPPLIED

No. 3585 — Tablets PLENDIL, 5 mg, are light red-brown, round convex tablets, with code MSD 451 on one side and PLENDIL on the other. They are supplied as follows:
NDC 0006-0451-28 unit dose packages of 100
NDC 0006-0451-58 unit of use bottles of 100
NDC 0006-0451-31 unit of use bottles of 30.
No. 3586 — Tablets PLENDIL, 10 mg, are red-brown, round convex tablets, with code MSD 452 on one side and PLENDIL on the other. They are supplied as follows:
NDC 0006-0452-28 unit dose packages of 100
NDC 0006-0452-58 unit of use bottles of 100
NDC 0006-0452-31 unit of use bottles of 30.

Storage

Store below 30°C (86°F). Keep container tightly closed. Protect from light.

MERCK SHARP & DOHME, Division of Merck & Co., INC.
West Point, Pa. 19486

A.H.F.S. Category: 24:04

Issued July 1991   DC7650202